Skin Care Collection:
150 DIY Natural Organic Beauty Secrets for Healthy, Glowing Skin

Homemade Deodorant

Introduction

I want to thank you and congratulate you for downloading the book "Homemade Deodorant: 30 Best Non-Toxic Organic Deodorant and Body Spray Recipes to Keep You Dry And Smelling Fresh All Day Long!"

This book contains proven steps and strategies on how to make your own deodorant, body sprays, and perfumes.

The fact is commercial deodorants are not what they used to be. They are full of chemicals, harmful additives, and dyes that have been proven to be carcinogens, meaning they can cause cancer. In addition, they are endocrine disruptors, so they make you more susceptible to hormone abnormalities, which can also lead to cancer.

The bottom line is that deodorant that you purchase from the store is not healthy for you, but you can make your own version that works just as well, and doesn't come with the added risk of breast cancer, liver disease, and many other terrible complications!

Find out how to make your own deodorant, body spray, and perfume throughout this book.

Chapter One – Why Use Organic Ingredients?

Deodorant is a habitual practice that just about no one actually thinks about. It's a convenient roll on liquid, spray or a traditional stick application. Its purpose is to make sure that when you lift up your arms, no one has the pleasant surprise of smelling something unpleasant. Deodorant is your defense against wet underarms and smelly armpits, but what's in the current deodorant you might be wearing?

In this chapter, we're going to go over some of the common ingredients found in the conventional deodorant you might be purchasing, and see if these odor and sweat blocking additives are what you really want stuck to your underarms all day.

Once you understand the ingredients in conventional deodorant, you'll know why you should use organic ingredients to make your own deodorant.

Aluminum

Aluminum is the main ingredient that's included in antiperspirant deodorants. This is a metal that's used to block your sweat glands, decreasing your capability to sweat by an average of twenty percent. The problem with this common metal is that it can cause serious health risks such as breast cancer and Alzheimer's disease.

Due to aluminum's main function being to block the sweat glands, what happens to all of your sweat? The underarms are closely linked to the lymph nodes, so this accumulation of toxins from your sweat not being perspired can potentially cause mayhem in your armpits. No amount of build-up of toxins in your body is good for you, and long-term build-up can cause cell mutation.

While the link between aluminum and breast cancer has controversial studies, it still convincing them with most breast cancer is developing in the upper outer quadrant of the breasts, which is the close a squadron to your armpit with lymph nodes are located, the long-term use of commercial deodorant with aluminum is factored into the formation of certain breast cancers.

In addition, women are more likely to shave under their arms, which mean excess aluminum is able to pass through this area more effectively. This could be the reason why breast cancer is more common amongst women.

Propylene Glycol

Another ingredient that's frequently used in deodorants is propylene glycol. Propylene glycol is a substance that is derived from petroleum and use to make a soft and silky consistency. It's a cheap ingredient that has a versatile function, and this is the reason it's so common in beauty products. Propylene glycol acts as a penetration enhancer, so if it's paired with harmful chemicals it will increase their absorption.

Recent studies have shown that propylene glycol is considered to be nontoxic to the body when it's ingested. It's eliminated from the body after a few hours, which is why it's considered nontoxic. However, there are reports of its potential toxicity being linked to issues such as:

- Cancer

- Developmental abnormalities

- Reproductive complications

- Endocrine complications

- Neurotoxicity

Propylene glycol has a single main concern beings that it's a skin sensitizer, which means it can cause allergic reactions such as irritant contact dermatitis, non-immunologic contact urticarial (hives), and allergic contact dermatitis.

Itching profusely under the arms can be very annoying, not to mention embarrassing.

Phthalates

This ingredient, also known as fragrance on the ingredient list, is a plasticizing chemical that's often used in many other beauty products due to their consistency and their capability to help dissolve some of the other ingredients.

The performance and the function of the ingredient seem to be more important to the conventional skin care brands than the quality and the safety of the ingredients.

This product helps your deodorant glide on smoothly, but what are the consequences of it being in your deodorant? It is worth having a temporary fix that could possibly cause a larger problem later on?

Phthalates are linked to many health issues and are considered endocrine disruptors. Once they are absorbed by your body, they act like estrogen, which not only conflict with hormonal function, but they also cause many other complications, such as:

- Decreased sperm count

- Infertility

- Prostate, breast, and ovarian cancer

- Lung, liver, and kidney damage

- Asthma

- Endometriosis

- Allergies

These are a probable human carcinogen and while the United States continues to regulate them, they're still very prevalent in many beauty products, including deodorants.

Sometimes, you might not consider the potential harm of a simple step of getting ready in the morning, but little do you know that your deodorant, antiperspirants, and your body sprays are all just another pitfall in an endless chemical burden of the conventional skin care products.

So skip the dangerous commercial deodorants, body sprays, perfumes, and mists, and try out some of the recipes in this book!

Chapter Two – Organic Deodorant Recipes

Homemade Deodorant with Shea Butter

Ingredients

- 3 Tbsp. Coconut Oil

- 2 Tbsp. Shea Butter

- 3 Tbsp. Baking Soda

- 2 Tbsp. Arrowroot Powder

- Essential Oils Of Your Choice

Directions

1. Melt the coconut oil and the Shea butter in a double boiler over medium heat until they're just melted. You want to combine in a quart sized glass mason jar with a lid instead and put this in a small saucepan of water until it's melted. This saves you a bowl and you can just designate this jar for this type of project and not need to wash it out. This can also be done in your microwave.

2. Remove this from the heat and add the arrowroot and the baking soda.

3. Mix it all together well.

4. Add the essential oils and then pour it all into a glass container to store it. It doesn't need to be refrigerated.

5. If you like, you can allow it to cool totally and put it into an old deodorant stick for easier usage, thought it could melt in the summer.

Take note this recipe can take a few hours to completely harden and the process can be sped up by putting it in the refrigerator for a few minutes.

Coconut Oil Homemade Deodorant Recipe

Ingredients

- 6 Tbsp. Coconut Oil

- ¼ C. Baking Soda

- ¼ C. Arrowroot Powder

- Essential Oils Of Your Choice

Directions

1. Mix the arrowroot powder and the baking soda together in a medium bowl.

2. Mash the oil with a fork until it's well incorporated.

3. Add the oils if you prefer them.

4. Store it in a small, glass jar or an old deodorant container.

Deodorant Bar Recipe

Ingredients

- ½ C. Coconut Oil

- ½ C. Shea Butter

- ½ C. Beeswax

- 1 Tsp. Vitamin E Oil

- 3 Tbsp. Baking Soda

- ½ C. Organic Arrowroot Powder

- 3 Capsules High Quality Probiotics

- 20 Drops Essential Oil Of Your Choice

Directions

1. Combine the coconut oil, shea butter and the beeswax in a double boiler or a glass bowl that's set over a smaller saucepan with an inch of water in it. You can also use a quart sized glass mason jar with a lid and put it in a small saucepan of hot water. This saves you the bowl and you can designate the jar for this type of project and not have to wash it out.

2. Turn the burner on and bring your water to a boil. Stir the ingredients continuously until they're melted and smooth.

3. Remove them from the heat and add the vitamin E oil, arrowroot powder, baking soda, probiotics, and the essential oils. Be sure the oil isn't too hot so the heat won't kill your probiotics. If you can touch it without being burnt, it's not too hot.

4. Gently stir it until all the ingredients are well combined.

5. If you want to make this into bars, then pour it into muffin tins or another mold that will hold liquid. If you are going to put it into an old deodorant container and use it like stick deodorant, then let the mix hard-

en for around twenty minutes. When it's around the consistency of peanut butter, use a spoon to scoop it into the tube and pack it down in. Then, allow the cup to stay off overnight to completely harden the deodorant before using it.

Homemade Deodorant for Sensitive Skin

Ingredients

- ¾ C. Cornstarch or Arrowroot Powder

- ¼ C. Baking Soda

- 6 Tbsp. Melted Coconut Oil

Directions

1. Combine the arrowroot powder or cornstarch with the baking soda.

2. Add four tablespoons of the coconut oil to the mix and mash it down with a fork until it's well combined. Keep adding the coconut oil until the deodorant reaches a consistency you like.

3. Transfer the mix to a jar that has a tight fitting lid.

4. To use the deodorant, apply a little under your arms with your fingertips as it's needed.

Homemade Deodorant Recipe for Sensitive Skin

Ingredients

* ¾ C. Cornstarch or Arrowroot Powder

* ¼ C. Diatomaceous Earth (Food Grade)

* 9 Tbsp. Melted Coconut Oil

Directions

1. Combine the arrowroot or cornstarch with the diatomaceous earth.

2. Add six tablespoons of melted oil and mix it up with a fork. Keep adding the oil until the deodorant has reached your desired consistency.

3. Then transfer to a jar that has a tight fitting lid and apply a small amount under your arms when it's needed.

All-Natural Homemade Deodorant Recipe

Ingredients

* ½ Tbsp. Baking Soda

* ⅛ C. Arrowroot Powder

* ⅛ C. Cocoa Butter

* ⅛ C. Shea Butter

* 5 Vitamin E Oil Drops

* 25-40 Drops Your Chosen Essential Oil

Directions

1. Using a Pyrex measuring glass, combine the shea butter and the cocoa butter.

2. Use a double boiler to heat the oils over medium heat until they are melted.

3. Remove them from the heat and stir in the baking soda and the arrowroot powder.

4. Stir in the vitamin E oil and your essential oils.

5. Carefully pour this mix into two ounce tins, filling them to the top, but making sure not to spill it over.

6. Put the lids on the container but don't press down to lock them. Just allow them to rest on the top to help prevent any dust from settling into the deodorant as it settles.

7. Let it completely cool and solidify, which can take six or more hours. Letting it sit overnight is best.

Homemade Deodorant

Ingredients

- ½ C. Coconut Oil
- ½ C. Baking Soda
- 40-60 Essential Oil Drops
- Empty Deodorant Container

Directions

1. Put the oil into a bowl.

2. Mix the baking soda into it.

3. Add the essential oil and mix well.

4. Store it in your deodorant container or in a glass jar.

Recipe for Homemade Summer Deodorant

Ingredients

- ¼ C. Cornstarch

- ¼ C. Baking Soda

- 3 Tbsp. coconut Oil

- 1 Tbsp. Beeswax, Grated

- 5 Tea Tree Oil Drops

- 5 Essential Oil Drops of Your choice

Directions

1. Start by melting the oil and the wax together in a double boiler. Rest a heat-proof bowl inside a saucepan that has an inch worth of water in the bottom. Heat it gently, stirring continuously, until the wax has melted.

2. Add the rest of the ingredients.

3. Stir it together. At this point, you will have a runny paste or slurry. This changes quickly.

4. Work quickly by pouring the paste into the empty deodorant container. By the end of this step, you might have to scrape the last bit of paste into the container and push it down, smoothing the top. That's how quickly it will begin to solidify.

Lemon Juice

Ingredients

- Lemon Juice

Directions

1. Many people like to use lemon as a natural deodorizer. Lemon juice contains citric acid that helps kill the odor-causing bacteria under your arms. Use a lemon slice on your armpits every morning. Remember, don't use lemon juice on any recently shaved areas, though!

Rubbing Alcohol

Ingredients

- Rubbing Alcohol
- Cotton Ball

Directions

1. Rubbing alcohol is another way to kill odor causing bacteria. It's inexpensive and very easy to use, too. You can just fill a spray bottle with

rubbing alcohol and spritz it under your arms, or you can use a cotton ball and gently dab it on. Adding an essential oil will make it into a pretty, scented spritzer, too.

Detoxifying Deodorant

Ingredients

- 5 Tbsp. Coconut Oil

- 3 Tbsp. Baking Soda

- 3 Tbsp. Arrowroot Powder

- 2 Tbsp. Bentonite Clay

- 20 Tea Tree Oil Drops

Directions

1. Put everything in a mixing bowl in the order that it's listed in. because coconut oil is a solid when it's at room temperature, it has to be heated to be able to mix it easily. With your clean hands, knead the mixture until everything makes a smooth paste. Then transfer this paste to a glass jar or a deodorant stick.

2. The paste will thicken after you let it cool at room temperature. To apply it, just rub your finger on the top of the paste and scoop out a little amount to rub on your underarms. The pate will melt right into the sick and absorb quickly.

All-Natural Coconut Deodorant

Ingredients

- ¼ C. Coconut Oil

- ⅛ C. Cornstarch

- ⅛ C. Arrowroot Powder

- Essential Oils of Your Choice

- 1 Tbsp. Baking Soda

Directions

1. Combine the oil, cornstarch, baking soda, and the arrowroot powder in a mixing bowl. When it's well combined, add in your essential oil a few drops at a time until you get to the scent you prefer.

2. Pour it into an empty deodorant container or just pour it into a small mason jar and refrigerator it for fifteen minutes. Remove it from the refrigerator and use it as you need it.

3. If you're using a mason jar, you'll need to chip out some little piece and then rub it onto your armpit. The deodorant melts and applies smoothly to your skin.

DIY Natural Deodorant Solid Recipe

Ingredients

- 2 Tbsp. Coconut Oil

- 1 Tbsp. Beeswax

- 1 Tbsp. Shea Butter

- 2 Tbsp. Arrowroot Powder

- 1 ½ Tbsp. Bentonite Clay

- 1 Tbsp. Baking Soda

- 2 Drops Citronella Essential Oil

- 2 Drops Lemongrass Essential Oil

- 2 Drops Tea Tree Essential Oil

Directions

1. In a double boiler, add the shea butter, coconut oil, and the wax. Bring it all to a boil over medium heat and stir until the wax and oils are melted.

2. Remove it from the heat and add in the bentonite clay, baking soda, arrowroot powder, and the essential oils. Mix it all well.

3. Pour the liquid into some silicone muffin molds or a five ounce container, such as an empty deodorant container.

4. Let it cool down and solidify for around two to three hours. The wax will help keep it solid so you can use it as a traditional deodorant.

Easy Deodorant

Ingredients

- ¼ C. Baking Soda

- ¼ C. Cornstarch or Arrowroot Powder

- 5 Tbsp. Coconut Oil

Directions

1. Combine the arrowroot powder and the baking soda together with a fork. Start with around four tablespoons of the oil and then add it to the baking soda mix. Work it into a paste.

2. Add the rest if you feel you need to.

3. You can store this in a small container or put it in an empty deodorant stick.

Vitamin E Deodorant

Ingredients

- 3 Tbsp. Shea Butter

- 2 Tbsp. Cornstarch

- 3 Tbsp. Baking Soda

- 2 Tbsp. Cocoa Butter

- 2 Vitamin E Caps

- Essential Oil of your choice

Directions

1. Melt everything but the oil together and stir it.

2. The mix in the oil and pour it into a container, and put the container in the refrigerator to let it set.

3. This recipe will fill a ¼ pint jar.

Chapter Three – Organic Body Spray Recipes

Vanilla and Ylang-Ylang Body Spray

Ingredients

- 18 Vanilla Oleoresin Drops
- 2 Ylang-Ylang Drops
- ¼ C. Witch Hazel with Alcohol

Directions

1. Mix everything together in a dark colored spray bottle and store it in a dark place.

Vanilla and Sweet Orange Body Spray

Ingredients

- 16 Vanilla Oleoresin Drops
- 4 Sweet Orange Essential Oil Drops
- ¼ C. Witch Hazel with Alcohol

Directions

1. Mix everything together in a dark colored bottle and store it in a dark place.

Vanilla and Coffee Body Spray

- 16 Vanilla Oleoresin Drops

- 4 Coffee Essential Oil Drops

- ¼ C. Witch Hazel with Alcohol

Directions

1. Mix everything together in a dark colored spray bottle and store it in a dark, cool place.

Vanilla Clove Body Oil Spray

Ingredients

- ¼ C. Almond Oil

- ½ tsp. Vanilla Extract or Essential Oil

- 3 Drops Clove Oil

- Spray Bottle

Directions

1. Combine the ingredients and pour it into a small spray bottle.

Orange Blossom Body Spray

Ingredients

- 1 oz. Filtered Water

- 90 Drops Orange Essential Oil

- ½ tsp. Vegetable Glycerine

Directions

1. Add everything to a small spray bottle, shake to combine and spritz onto your skin. Be sure to rub it in.

Bohemian Patchouli Body Spray

Ingredients

- 1 oz. filtered water

- ⅛ tsp. Tunisian Patchouli Essential Oil

- ½ tsp. Vegetable Glycerine

Directions

1. Mix it together in a small, glass spray bottle and shake it well. Shake it before you use it.

Citrus Energy Natural Body Spray

Ingredients

- 1 oz. Distilled Water

- ½ oz. Witch Hazel with Alcohol

- ½ oz. Vegetable Glycerin

- 10 Grapefruit Essential Oil Drops

- 4 Lime Essential Oil Drops

- 4 Lemon Essential Oil Drops

Directions

1. Mix everything together in a small glass bottle and shake it well. Shake it before every use.

Orange Vanilla Natural Body Spray

Ingredients

- 1 oz. Distilled Water

- ½ oz. Witch Hazel with Alcohol

- ½ oz. Vegetable Glycerin

- ⅛ tsp. Vanilla Extract

- 10 Drops Orange Essential Oil

Directions

1. Mix it all together in a small glass bottle and shake it well. Shake it before every use.

Purifying Linen and Body Spray

Ingredients

- 1 C. Water
- 120 Drops Essential Oil
    - 20 Drops Peppermint
    - 40 Drops Lemon
    - 40 Drops Eucalyptus
- Dark Brown Spray Bottle (Glass)

Directions

1. Pour the water into the bottle
2. Add the essential oils.
3. Shake before you use it.

Moisturizing Body Spray

Ingredients

- ¼ C. Distilled Water

- 1 ½ tsp. Vegetable Glycerin

- 1 tsp. Grapeseed Oil

- 5 Drops Vitamin E Oil

- 10 Drops Essential Oil

Directions

1. Combine all the ingredients and carefully pour them into a small spray bottle, around three ounces. Shake it well before you use it.

2. Spray it liberally on your body as it's needed, especially after you shower. Rub it into your skin.

Lemon, Lavender, and Vanilla Body Spray

Ingredients

- 1 Glass Spray Bottle, 4 oz.

- 3 ½ oz. Vodka

- 5 Drops Lemon essential Oil

- 15 Drops Lavender Essential Oil

- 30 Drops Vanilla Essential Oil

Directions

1. Combine everything into a spray bottle and shake it well before using it.

Woodland Body Spray

Ingredients

- 4 Drops Spruce Essential Oil

- 2 Drops Cedarwood Essential Oil

- 2 Drops Fir Needle Essential Oil

- 1 Drop Bergamot Essential Oil

- 1 Drop Vetiver Essential Oil

- 1 tsp. Jojoba Oil

Directions

1. Add all the essential oils into the glass bottle and mix the oils with a wooden skewer or by shaking it gently.

2. Add the oil and shake it again.

3. Add more essential oil if you want it to be a little stronger.

Cucumber, Aloe Body Mist

Ingredients

- 1 Squeeze Lemon

- 1 Cucumber

- 1 tsp. Aloe Vera Gel

- 1 Tbsp. Rosewater

Directions

1. Peel the cucumber and dice it into pieces. Put them in a blender and pulse it on high for around a minute.

2. Cover a bowl with some cheese cloth and then strain the juice into the bowl.

3. Add the rest of the ingredients to the bowl and mix it thoroughly.

4. Transfer the mix to a spray bottle and you're done. You can add a little distilled water if you feel you need to dilute it a bit.

5. Store it in the refrigerator so it doesn't spoil. It'll last around a week.

Tropical Body Mist

Ingredients

- 1 oz. Distilled Water

- 10ml Rose Hydrosol

- 2 tsp. Vanilla Extract

- 1 tsp. Vodka

- 1 Tbsp. Vegetable Glycerin

- 1 Tbsp. Coconut Oil

- 5 Grapefruit Essential Oil drops

- 15 Neroli Essential Oil Drops

Directions

1. Begin by filling the spray bottle with some lukewarm distilled water and the hydrosol.

2. Add the vegetable glycerin slowly and then add the coconut oil. Use a wooden skewer to mix the two.

3. Make sure you're happy with the scent thus far and the consistency.

4. Then add the essential oils and close the spray bottle. Shake it well.

5. Let it rest a few hours before you use it the first time.

6. Always shake it well to make sure all the ingredients are mixed well.

Vanilla Cardamom Mist

Ingredients

- 6 Cardamom Seeds

- ½ C. Water

- 1 tsp. Vanilla Extract

Directions

1. Crack the seeds to expose their pods.

2. Put the bits of cardamom into a saucepan with the water and bring it to a boil. Remove it from the heat.

3. Let the cardamom water cool totally.

4. Transfer the scented water to a spray bottle.

5. Add the vanilla, seal the spray bottle, and shake it.

6. Adjust the amount of vanilla extract to your preference and store in a cool, dry place.

Grapefruit Mist

Ingredients

- 10 Drops Grapefruit Essential Oil

- Vodka

- Distilled Water

- Glass Spray Bottle

Directions

1. Fill the glass bottle up around two-thirds of the way with the vodka and add a few drops of the essential oil before you fill the bottle up the rest of the way with the distilled water.

Chapter Four – Organic Perfume Recipes

Solid Perfume

Ingredients

- 1 ½ Tbsp. Beeswax

- 1 ½ Tbsp. Olive Oil

- 40 Drops Essential Oil of your choice

Directions

1. Fill up a pan with half a cup of water and put it on the burner. Turn the burner heat to medium. Put the wax beads into a heatproof glass bowl and put it inside the pan. When it's melted, mix in the oil. Let it melt for another five minutes.

2. Remove the glass owl from the pan and quickly stir in the essential oil. Pour this into its final container.

3. The essential oils will smell strong in the beginning, but they will fade over time.

4. To use the solid perfume, wipe it on the interior of your wrist for a clean scent that'll last all day.

California Citrus Sunshine

Ingredients

- 1 Tbsp. Jojoba Oil

- 2 Tbsp. Grain Alcohol

- 7 Drops Sweet Orange Essential Oil

- 7 Drops Grapefruit Essential Oil

- 7 Drops Peppermint Essential Oil

- 7 Drops Lavender Essential Oil

- 1 Tbsp. Distilled Water

Directions

1. Begin by adding the jojoba to a glass container and then add the alcohol. It's important to use glass and not plastic.

2. Add the essential oils in the order they were listed in on the ingredients list.

3. Add the distilled water using a dropper.

4. Mix the ingredient well and transfer them to a dark container for forty-eight hours up to six weeks. The longer it sits, the stronger the scent is going to be.

5. Transfer it to a pretty perfume bottle after it's reached your desired scent.

Solid Shimmer Perfume

Ingredients

- 2 tsp. almond oil

- Essential oils of your choice

- 1 oz. beeswax

Directions

1. To make the solid perfume, combine the almond oil with the essential oils until you reach your desired scent.

2. The melt the wax and in a small glass in your microwave and add the oil mix. Stir it to combine it. Then pour it into a small mold to let it harden.

3. Add a small amount of shimmery eye shadow to give it some sparkle.

How to make Solid Essential Oil Perfume

Ingredients

- 1 Tbsp. beeswax

- 1 ½ Tbsp. Jojoba Oil

- 70 Drops Essential Oil

Directions

1. Grate or chop the beeswax finely and put it in the milk jug. Measure the oil into a small glass and then add the essential oil drops to your desired scent.

2. Melt the wax by filling the saucepan with about an inch of water, and then putting a glass container in the water. Put the beeswax into the

glass and avoid spilling any water into the glass. Bring the water to a simmer and melt the wax.

3. As soon as it's done, add the oil and stir it with a wooden skewer until it's well combined. Carefully remove it from the hot water. The glass is going to be hot, so use a cloth to protect your hands.

4. Quickly pour the wax into containers and let it rest for half an hour or until it's cooled down. To use it, just rub the wax surface with your fingertips and then rub it on your wrists and neck.

Lavender Vanilla Mist

Ingredients

- ½ C. Vodka
- 2 Tbsp. Vegetable Glycerin
- 1 C. Dried Lavender Flowers
- 2 Vanilla Beans
- 10 Drops Vanilla Extract
- 15 Drops lavender Essential Oil

Directions

1. Slice the vanilla bean open with a sharp knife.
2. Put the beans and the flowers in a large glass jar with a lid.
3. Pour the vodka into the jar and secure the lid.

4. Let the mix infuse for a week.

5. Strain and discard your vanilla beans and your lavender flowers.

6. Add the lavender essential oil, the glycerin, and the vanilla extract to the reserved liquids and stir it well.

7. Replace the lid and let it age for four to six weeks.

8. Strain the perfume once again through a paper filter and then transfer it to a decorate spray bottle.

Midnight Perfume

Ingredients

- 2 Tbsp. Jojoba Oil or Grape Seed Oil

- 6 Tbsp. Vodka

- 2 ½ Tbsp. Distilled Spring Water

- Funnel

- Coffee Filter

- Essential Oils

    - 15 Drops Clove Oil

    - 6 Drops Cedarwood Oil

    - 9 Drops lavender Oil

- 2 Dark Colored Glass Bottles

- Decorate Perfume Bottle

Directions

1. Start by cleaning the bottles, either in the dishwasher on the hottest setting or with some hot, soapy water. Put the bottles on a rimmed baking sheet and dry them in an oven set at 230 degrees Fahrenheit. Remove them from the oven when they're totally dry.

2. Put a lid on one of them and set it aside until you need it, which will anywhere from two days to six weeks later.

3. Put the carrier oil in one of your bottles.

4. Then add the essential oils.

5. Add the vodka.

6. Put the lid on top of the bottle and shake it well for several minutes.

7. Let it rest for forty-eight hours to six weeks.

8. The scent changes over time, becoming its strongest around six weeks.

9. Check it weekly and once you're happy with the scent, add two tablespoons of spring water to it and shake it well for a minute.

10. Put the coffee filter into the funnel and transfer your perfume from the bottle it's in to the perfume bottle. Label it and store it in a cool, dark place.

Citrus Lavender

Ingredients

- 2 tsp. Beeswax

- 48 Drops Essential Oils

- - ○ 12 Drops Sweet Orange Essential Oil

  - ○ 12 Drops Lemon Essential Oil

  - ○ 12 Drops lavender Essential Oil

  - ○ 12 Drops Bergamot Essential Oil

- 2 tsp. Jojoba Oil

- ½ oz. Tin

Directions

1. It's a good idea to blend the oils first before you begin working with the beeswax because it will harden very quickly.

2. Put all your essential oils into one cup so you can pour them into the beeswax mix when it's time.

3. You can play around with the amount of oil that you use and try to substitute different ones if you don't like the ones that were listed.

4. You can also use sweet almond oil for the carrier oil, too.

5. In another cup from the essential oils, measure out two teaspoons of the oil of your choice.

6. Measuring out the oil ahead of time saves you from having to rush around once the wax has melted.

7. If you have pellets of wax, then measure out two teaspoons of them into a small saucepan over medium to low heat.

8. If you have a block of wax, then you should grate off around a tablespoon of wax and then melt them in the pot. Then measure to make sure you have two teaspoons.

9. After you measure, you may find you have to heat the wax up again in the pan a few more seconds because it might begin to harden after you pour it into a measuring spoon.

10. Once you have the two teaspoons of the melted beeswax, add the carrier oil to it and stir it around until they're both combined.

11. Then take the pot off the burner and very quickly add the essential oils. Stir until they are well combined.

12. As quickly as you can, pour the mix into the container.

13. Cover it and allow it to rest ten minutes before you enjoy it.

Conclusion

Thank you again for downloading this book!

I hope this book was able to help you to learn how to make your own deodorant.

The next step is to gather up your ingredients and start cooking!

Finally, if you enjoyed this book, please take the time to share your thoughts and post a review on Amazon. It'd be greatly appreciated!

Thank you and good luck!

Essential Oils

Introduction

If you have spent any amount of time online, you know that it is important to watch what you are putting in or on your body. You know that there are medications and supplements that are meant to help your health in a variety of ways, but then you read that you should avoid a whole list of items that are then found in the supplements you are using.

So what do you do?

You know that you want to do the best thing for your health and your body, but what are you supposed to do when the very things you are supposed to use for your health end up being full of the very things you try to avoid.

You think of how you want to do what is best for your health, for your family, and for the planet, but you don't think you can do this if you are supporting the synthetic products that are on the shelves today.

This is a common feeling that a lot of people share, and thankfully the number one solution to this problem is also the solution to your health concerns. Essential oils are entirely natural, free of harmful synthetic chemicals, and can be used in more ways than any synthetic medication you could imagine.

You have a headache, you want to relax, and you want to settle the house down at the end of the day.

You don't want to turn to the synthetic medications that are full of warnings and things to watch for, but what do you do?

Essential oils is the answer. You can diffuse a few drops in a diffuser, you can apply a few drops directly to your skin, or you can even add certain kinds to tea, and you get the same great results.

Calm, quiet tranquility fills your home, and you feel better.

That's just the beginning. The more familiar you get with essential oils, the more you will be able to treat the ailments that arise, and the more natural you can live.

So are you ready to jump into the world of essential oils?

Naturally.

Chapter 1 – Getting Started

There is a lot of excitement when you start out in this journey, but before you just dive in and spread oils on everything, I want to get you started on the right track. This means you need to know what you are doing from the beginning.

You can't just toss essential oils around and see what happens, you have to know what each oil does, and how to use them for your particular symptoms. This is something you can use both ways. You can use this knowledge to use the right oil for your particular ailment, and you can avoid the oils that won't help you or potentially make you feel worse.

On the other hand, if you know what oils create different results, you will be able to set up your home with a lot of preventative aspects, meaning you won't get sick as often or feel the stress to begin with.

So, let's dive in and learn the facts about essential oils, how to use them, and what oils work well with each other.

Knowledge is an effective weapon.

The Wonder Oils

While each section you find is going to have its own list of oils, there are a few oils that seem to stand out from the rest. Yes, there are going to be times when you need to treat something specific, and you will need an equally specific oil to get the job done, but on the other hand, you are going to see a few oils show up time and time again, no matter what the ailment happens to be.

These are the oils I would like to refer to as the Wonder Oils, because there are so many ways using these oils can make your life better.

They are good for the specifics, and they are good for the broad categories.

Whether you are dealing with aches, pains, illness, insomnia, or want to promote things such as peace, tranquility, focus, happiness, and better relationships, these are the oils you always want to have on hand.

Peppermint

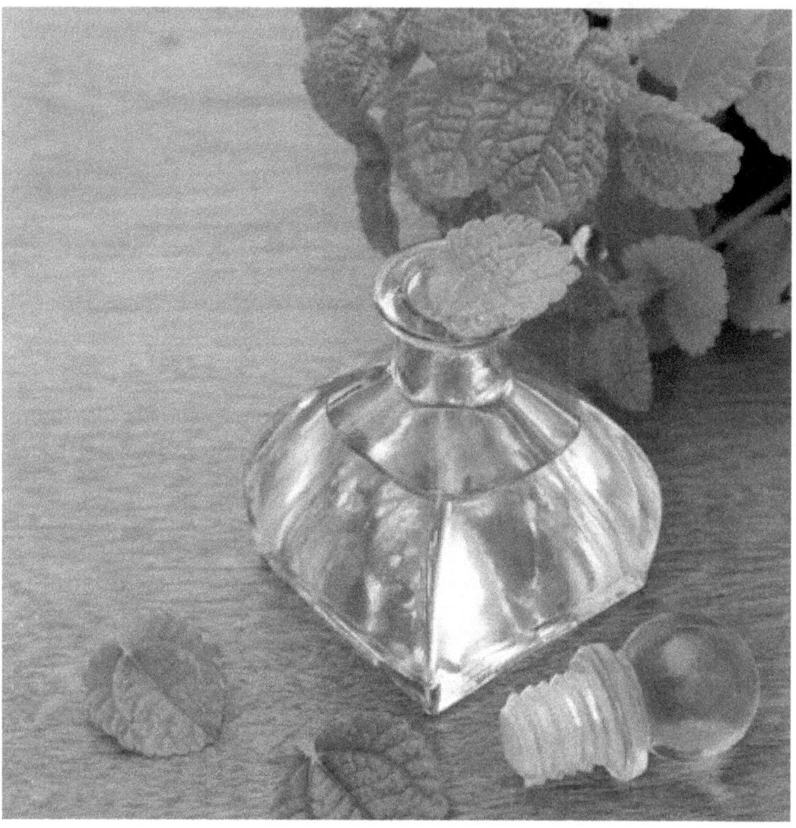

https://www.google.com/search?
q=peppermint+essential+oil&espv=2&biw=1366&bih=623&source=lnms&tbm=isch&sa=X&ved=0ahUKEwittoLvqo-
LNAhVDM1IKHfg9BSMQ_AUIBygC#imgrc=ahsC9-zCsT8oEM%3A

While many of us may associate this scent and taste with the holidays, there are a few things you need to know about this delightful oil that has nothing to do with Christmas trees or Santa Clause.

Peppermint oil has a light, fresh scent that blends exceptionally well with most other oils. It can be diffused for aroma therapy, applied topically on various aches and pains, and it can be enjoyed internally if it is highly diluted in water or tea. This oil is going to ease pains, clear your mind, and make you feel better and at peace.

It is abundantly available... you can purchase it not only online but in a variety of health and wellness stores to even large chain department stores. This oil truly is a wonder worker, and I suggest you keep plenty of it on hand at all times.

Lavender

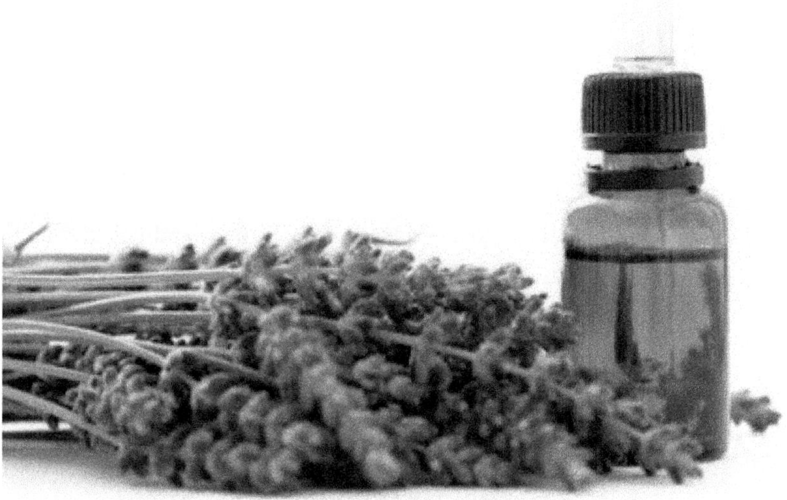

The floral scent of lavender is soothing to the mind, body, and soul. You would be amazed at how many people there are who think they don't like floral scents, but gravitate toward lavender.

Certainly among the best of the best, lavender is easily considered a Wonder Oil.

This oil is like peppermint in regards to the fact it will ease many of your life's ailments. Whether you are tense, stressed, or unable to sleep, a few drops of this oil spread across your forehead, blended into your bath water, or diffused in your bedroom is going to ease all of that tension that has built up and help you not only fall asleep, but stay asleep.

When you realize you can't become dependent on it, but you can use it as freely as you like, you are going to realize even more why you should keep this on hand at all times.

Make a space in your cabinet to house your lavender, peppermint, and tea tree oils, and there are few things you will face that you won't be able to handle.

Tea tree

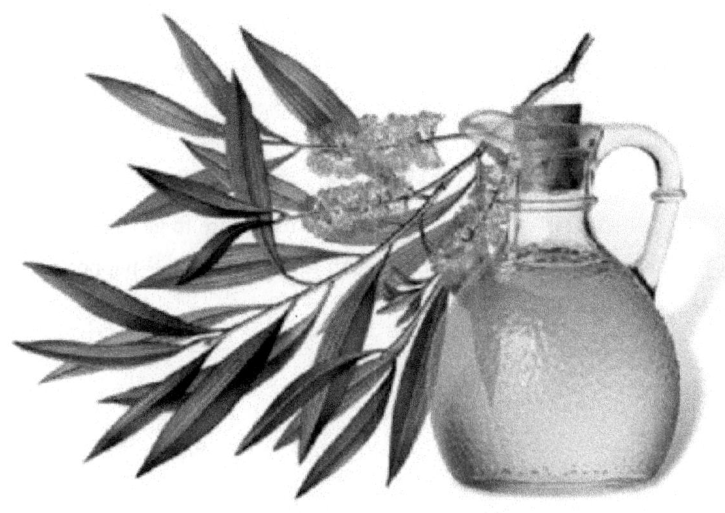

https://www.google.com/search?
q=tea+tree+oil&espv=2&biw=1366&bih=623&source=lnms&tbm=isch&sa=X&ved=0ahUKEwjR2YiQq4LNAhVIM-
FIKHT7rCgkQ_AUIBygC#imgrc=wfzRemDWCYN4oM%3A

When it comes to physical ailments and imperfections, few things are going to do more for you than tea tree oil. While this oil has a strong, somewhat overwhelming scent, the benefits it does for your skin are far beyond the strong scent it holds.

Tea tree oil is a natural antiseptic. You can apply it to scrapes, cuts, and even acne and it will heal and clear up the imperfection. Excellent for hair, skin, and even sore throats and coughs, this oil is best diffused into the air for aroma therapy or mixed with a carrier oil and applied topically.

If you want to lighten the scent of this Wonder Oil, you can blend it with less offensive oils such as lavender, rose, or lemon. Another terrific benefit that comes with tea tree oil is that it is even more abundant than peppermint or lavender. You can purchase large vials of the purest form online or in health food stores, and it doesn't cost nearly as much as some of the more exotic oils do.

This oil's benefits far outweigh the scent, so make sure to get a large vial of it and keep it up in your cabinet along with the lavender and peppermint. You will be so glad you did.

Chapter 2 – The Best of the Blends

You may only be experiencing one feeling, or you may want to promote a singular feeling, in which case you only need to choose the oil or oils that you enjoy. There are going to be times, however, when you need to address more than one problem at a time, or when you want to create a blend of energy in your home.

To do this, you need to combine oils in properly to get the desired effect.

Thankfully, blending oils is not only easy, it is encouraged to create the best fragrances and optimum results, so you won't have any problem at all finding the right blend for your needs.

The trick to getting the best of the blends is to know how to blend the oils yourself

If you get online, you are going to find that there are plenty of blends all ready to go. The supplier puts them together and sells them as a blend, usually under the name of what you need it for.

For example, you can purchase an oil blend from Doterra called "On Guard". It is an immunity support oil, but if you look closer at it, you will see that it is, in fact, a blend of the everyday oils you have on hand such as wild orange, clove bud, cinnamon, eucalyptus, and rosemary.

While there is a lot of convenience to purchasing the oil already blended, you are going to find that you will save a lot of money, and get a lot more of the product if you purchase the oils separately and blend them yourself.

Wait, purchasing all of those oils separately isn't going to be inexpensive… the blend is a lot cheaper to buy as it is

Yes, that may be true, but if you think about it, if you purchase the ingredients separately, not only do you get enough to make the blend yourself, but you also get the extra oils left over to put to other use.

This is going to come in handy if you want to have the immunity support, as well as treat any ailment you already have, or simply to set some aside until you need it again. You see, when you are blending the oils yourself, you always have a lot of each on hand, simply because you only use a few drops of each one when you do use it.

So that brings us to the actual blending aspect.

When you blend the oils yourself, make sure you look at the total number of drops you are going to be using at the end result. If you are making enough to save some, keep the ratios the same, but if you are only mixing one time use at a time, watch out for how much you are actually using.

What this means is that if you are going to use the oils to make the equivalent to Doterra's On Guard, you need to realize that the 2 drops you use from that bottle are 2 blended drops.

I know that sounds confusing at first, but think about it this way. If you are mixing in the On Guard into your tea to sip on, you only need 1 or 2 drops to do it. All of those oils I listed that create this blend come together in those 2 drops you put into your tea.

If you were to take each of those drops and place only 1 drop each in your tea separately, then you will end up with 5 or 6 drops, which is simply too much to ingest at one time. If you put this all in your tea at once, you will run into problems from overdosing on the oils.

To get around this, you need to cut back on the amount of oils you are using in your tea, or (better yet) blend them all separately then take 2 drops of what you have blended. The most important thing you need to remember when it comes to essential oils is that you can overdose, and too much of some of them can be toxic.

Keep small jar glasses on hand, or purchase some of your own vials to store the extra oils you blend. This is going to keep them safe until you need them again, and help you stay on track with the proper dosage of the oils.

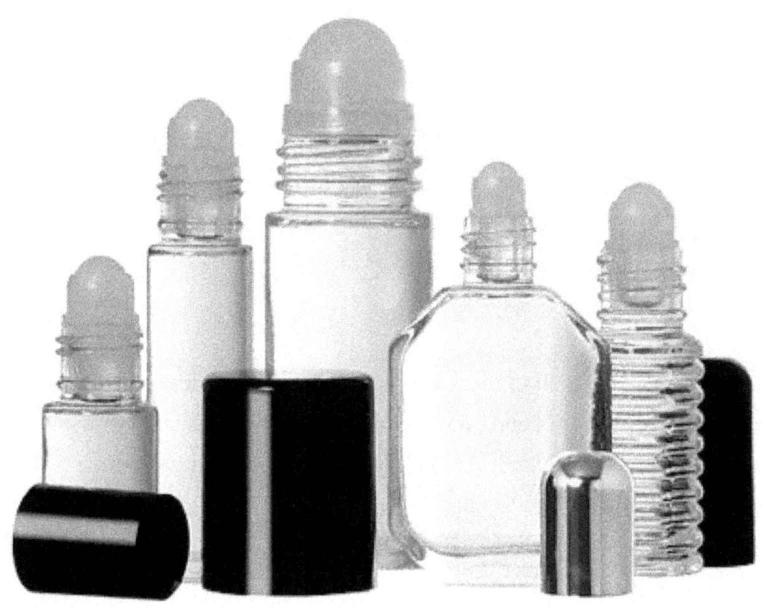

Small vials that have the drop lid are available online, or you can even get them locally at a number of stores. One of the major benefits to mixing your own blends in your own bottles is that you get to then choose the bottles you want to use as well.

This means you can create your own mists, roll ons, or drop bottles to suit your own taste, and keep them on hand where you want them. Say you want to take an anti-stress blend to work with you? No problem!

Purchase a roll on dispenser, mix up your favorite blend or just use your favorite anti-stress oil, fill your roll on dispense, and toss it in your purse. No matter where your day goes you will have your instant anti-stress mechanism at just an arm's length away, and your day is going to go so much better.

When you are creating your own blends, start with the desired effect you want your blend to have, and move on from there.

For example, if you want a blend that is going to help you sleep, but you also want to relieve tension and stress besides, start with the lavender. You want there to be more lavender in this blend than anything else, so I would recommend starting with 10 or 12 drops of this oil.

Then, pick the other oils you want. Peppermint is great for stress relief, so choose this one next, but don't put in the same amount. Perhaps 6 or 7 drops to suit your own taste.

What you want to keep in mind is that you want to use the most of your main focus, then add in the secondary oils as secondary benefits. Once you have this down, you can make any blend you want for any use you want.

Get creative!

Chapter 3 – Oils by Symptoms or Desired Effect

There are times when you are looking through the oils to see what they do, but there are also times when you feel a certain way and you want to find the oils that make it better.

What I mean by this is that you may enjoy the smell of rose oil and lavender oil, so you diffuse this in your home often. You are going to gain the amazing benefits that come from diffusing this oil... which means you are going to feel calm, relaxed, open, etc... but this doesn't help when you are suffering from a headache.

So, if you happen to have some sort of ailment (a headache, a stomach ache, a tooth ache), you need to know which oils to use specifically for these problems.

Here are oils separated into categories based on the symptoms you feel.

You can use one of the oils in the category, or you can mix and match as you please to take care of many of your symptoms.

Body Aches and Pains

Body aches and pains are annoying as well as debilitating. When you feel any of these symptoms, you know you want to get better as soon as possible.

I suggest for any of the oils or oil blends you use here, mix a few drops with a carrier oil and massage onto the aching area.

You can also add 10 to 12 drops into a warm bath and soak your pain away.

Headaches

Eucalyptus

Lavender

Peppermint

Stomach aches

Peppermint

Ginger

Roman chamomile

Melissa

Star anise

Grapefruit

Spearmint

Cardamom

Coriander

Fennel

Aniseed

Joint pain and stiffness

Sweet marjoram

Chamomile

Rosemary

Peppermint

Eucalyptus

Muscle cramps

Peppermint

Lemongrass

Basil

Vetiver

Sage

Cypress

Grapefruit

Rosemary

Natural Cold and Flu Remedies

When it comes to treating the cold and flu, I suggest you use a diffuser next to your bed or couch. The oils will fill the air and the aroma therapy will clear the illness right out.

If you are dealing with specific aches such as a sore throat, cough, or headache, you may also mix the oils of your choice with a carrier oil and massage it into the infected area, or add a drop or two to tea and sip on it.

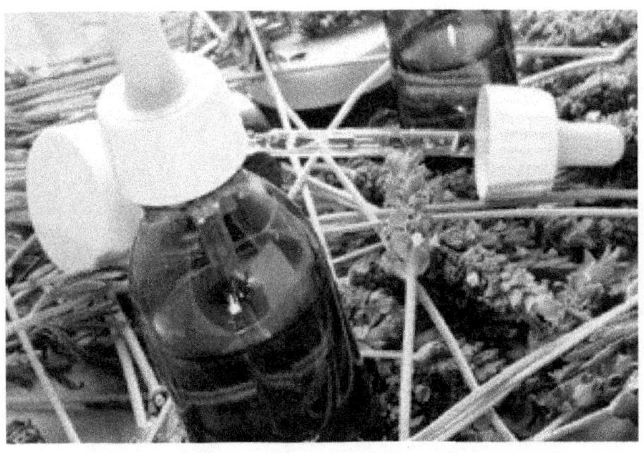

https://www.google.com/search?q=essential+oil+skin+care&espv=2&biw=1366&bih=623&site=webhp&source=lnms&tbm=isch&sa=X&ved=0ahUKEwj2qvG1qYLNAhUNSFIKHSunCKIQ_AUIBygC#imgrc=Bh2o8B1JeDrWnM%3A

Colds

Lavender

Eucalyptus

Thyme

Rosemary

Garlic

Sandalwood

Lemon

Chamomile

Peppermint

Sore Throat

Eucalyptus

Oregano

Sage

Tea tree

Ginger

Peppermint

Cough

Lavender

Peppermint

Lemongrass

Frankincense

Lemon

Stress

No matter what kind of job you work or what kind of life you live, you are going to deal with a level of stress.

To rid your mind and body of that stress, I strongly suggest you use these oils or any blend of these oils in a diffuser, or add 10 to 12 drops into your hot bath water before you soak in the tub.

Tension

Helichrysum

Peppermint

Spearmint

Roman chamomile

Eucalyptus

Lavender

Insomnia

Lavender

Roman chamomile

Sweet marjoram

Vetiver

Ylang ylang

Anxiety

Basil

Clary sage

Bergamot

Frankincense

Ylang ylang

Marjoram

Peppermint

The Air of the House is the Mood of the Home

They say prevention is the best cure, and if you set up your home to be a safe haven, you are going to skip out on a lot of stressful symptoms that pop up in day to day life.

Use these oils in diffusers around your home. Diffusers aren't expensive and they are easy to maintain.

Prevent ailments and issues and promote peace and health with these oils blended into the air of your home at all times.

The Essentials you will need:

To promote tranquility

Chamomile

Roman chamomile

Lavender

Cedar wood

To promote happiness

Orange

Rose

Jasmine

Ginger

Cloves

Sandalwood

Petitgrain

Frankincense

Lemon

Geranium

To promote energy

Black pepper

Bergamot

Grapefruit

Peppermint

Rosemary

Thyme

Lemon

Basil

Fennel

To promote peace

Tangerine

Orange

Patchouli

Ylang ylang

Cassia

Davana

German chamomile

Cistus

Lavender

Lemon

Chapter 4 – The Practical Side of Things

In life there are far more things we want to address and take care of besides mood and colds. You want beautiful hair, you want to lose weight or maintain a weight loss. Your teenagers want clear skin and you want to avoid or get rid of the wrinkles that somehow appeared around your mouth and eyes.

Sure, it's great to know how to address a headache or sleeplessness, but once you know how to also get rid of such things as acne, wrinkles, and oily hair, you are going to be completely taken care of in your oil usage.

That is why I have included this chapter, so you know exactly what you can use to treat or prevent those physical imperfections you don't want to have to deal with any longer.

And when you combine the fact you get to save money as well as save your skin from harmful chemicals, you have a complete win, and everyone wants to have that.

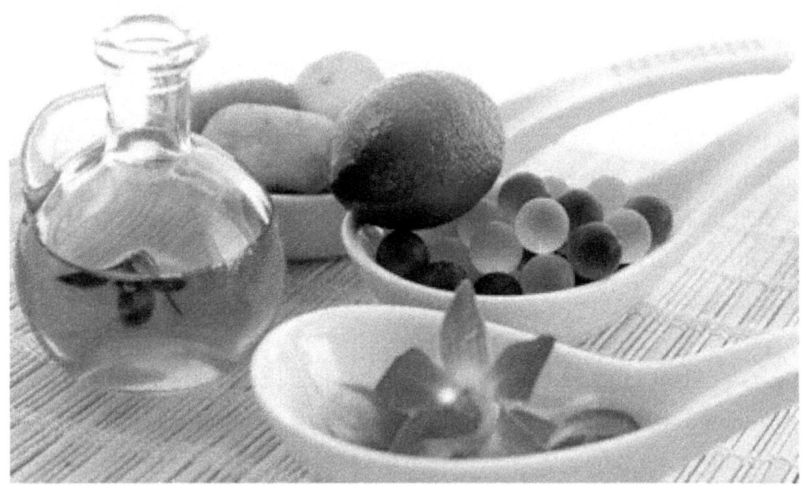

https://www.google.com/search?
q=essential+oil+skin+care&espv=2&biw=1366&bih=623&site=webhp&source=lnms&tbm=isch&sa=X&ved=0ah-
UKEwj2qvG1qYLNAhUNSFIKHSunCKIQ_AUIBygC#imgrc=Bh2o8B1JeDrWnM%3A

People of all ages across the globe spend hundreds and thousands of dollars each year on various skin care products. Each of the products claim they are going to do the magic trick, but most of them end up not working anyway.

Not to mention these products are full of chemicals you don't want on your skin. Using essential oils are always a better choice, and I promise you that you are going to see better results using these than you ever did with store products.

To use these, mix with your face soap, moisturizer, or with a carri-er oil and apply directly to the spot you want to focus on.

How to get rid of acne

Jojoba

Lavender

Tea tree

Orange

Frankincense

Get rid of those wrinkles!

Myrrh

Frankincense

Rose

Carrot seed

Lavender

Geranium

Sandalwood

Minimize the appearance of pores and say goodbye to freckles

Lemon

Tea tree

Lemongrass

Carrot seed

Geranium

Frankincense

For the Hair

Many commercials proudly proclaim that your hair is as unique as you, but you don't find this to be a good thing when you can't find any product that does what you need it to do.

Here are the oils you want to turn to based on what you need for your hair. Blend a few drops in with your shampoo and wash as you normally would.

The results are real, and you are going to love them.

The best oily hair treatment

Lavender

Cedar wood

Peppermint

Frankincense

Sage

Basil

Clary sage

Juniper

Hair growth oils

Thyme

Lavender

Rosemary

Moisture for the dry hair

Clary sage

Lemon

Thyme

Tea tree

Cedar wood

Weight Loss and Weight Management

It seems that majority of people want to lose weight, but once they do, it is a struggle to keep it off. If you bring in these oils, you are going to see the weight melt away, as well as keep it off for good.

I suggest you use a diffuser for these oils, or that you highly dilute a drop or two into a tall glass of water. The results are real, entirely natural, and not even remotely dangerous.

You really can lose that weight for good, and enjoy the results, knowing they are going to last.

Essential weight loss

Lemon

Grapefruit

Cypress

Ginger

Peppermint

Cinnamon

Garlic

Perfect weight management

Grapefruit

Tangerine

Lemon

Spearmint

Ocotea

Cinnamon bark

Thieves

And, of course…. Peppermint

I'm sure you saw the overlap I mentioned in chapter 1 of all the ways you can use the top 3 oils, but I do strongly urge you to go out and get as many oils as you can find. They have dozens for sale on Amazon, or you can look into the other private suppliers that are around both online and locally.

No matter where you decide to get your essential oils, the important thing you need to remember is to check that they are pure. A pure essential oil is going to come in a dark bottle, as this is the best way to store them. The liquid itself is going to be strongly scented, and have an oily appearance just by looking at it.

If you get your oils from reputable sources, you have nothing to worry about, so just go through somewhere you trust, and make sure it says on the label that it is 100% pure before you buy.

Chapter 5 – The Tricks of the Trade: How to Use Essential Oils

You can know all kinds of things about essential oils, whether it be which ones are best for certain symptoms, what blends smell the best, or what kind of oils you want to avoid in various situations, but all of this is just head knowledge unless you know how to take them from the vial and put them into your life.

There are a number of different methods that people use when it comes to essential oils.

The most common are:

1. Diffusing

2. Applying topical

3. Taking internally

Let's take a moment now to look at each one, and you can decide which method you prefer for yourself, or what combination of methods you want to use. Some people choose one, others combine one or two, then there are those that use all three, the great thing about essential oils and knowing how to use them is that you can do what you want, when you want it.

Diffusing

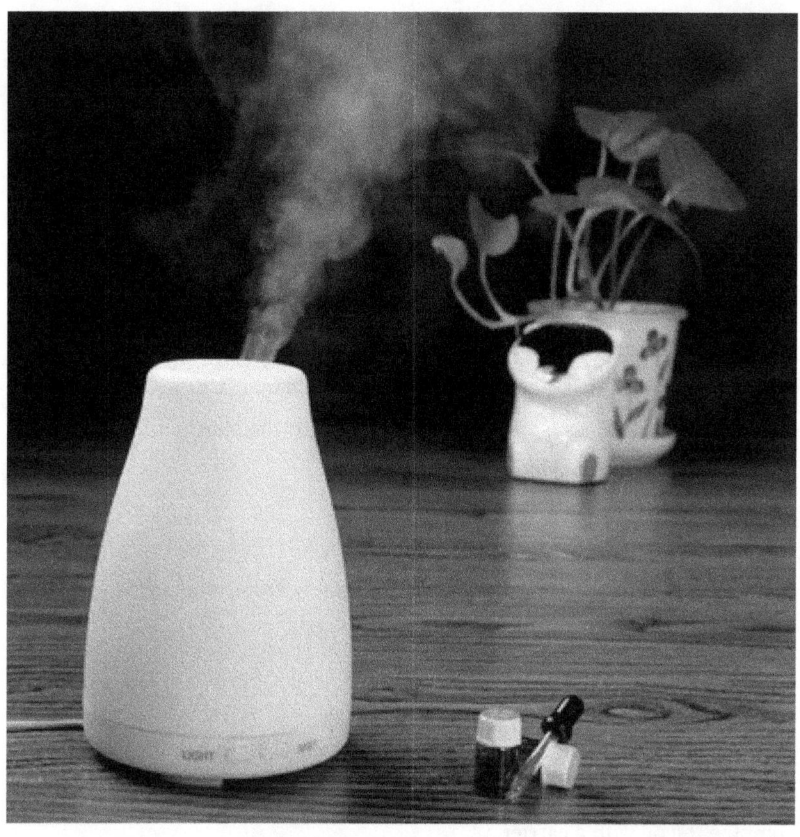

The most common method of using essential oils is diffusing. To do this, you purchase a diffuser, fill it with water (the amount of water varies with the diffuser you purchase), and add a few drops of oil.

If you know the specific symptom you want to treat, you put in the oil or blend of oils into the diffuser, plug it in, and let it fill the air with a delightful smelling mist. The aroma therapy treats the ailment, and makes your house smell incredible.

Topical use

Another prevalent method is applying the oil topically. When you do this, you still choose the oil you want based on the symptoms that are at hand. For example, you know that peppermint helps with stomach aches and lavender helps with restlessness, so if you are dealing with the stomach flu, a blend of these two oils will help a lot.

To apply topically, you are only going to use a few drops total, perhaps 2 drops of each oil.

Now, many oils are harsh applied directly to your skin, so you need to be careful with the oils you are using. The best way to prevent any skin irritation is to combine the oil with a carrier oil.

Carrier oils are mild oils that can be applied liberally to any part of your body, they are usually common oils such as coconut, sunflower, olive oil, or even vegetable oil if you are in a pinch.

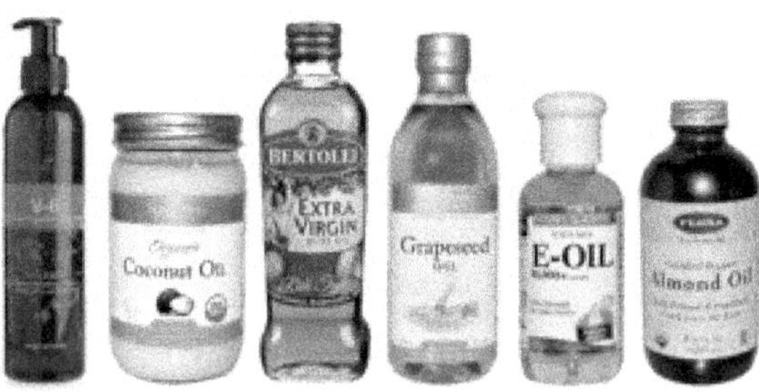

The best ratio I have found with the essential oil and the carrier oil is to combine a few drops of the essential oil with half a tablespoon of the carrier oil. Spread this on the part that is ailing (massage it into your forehead, onto your stomach, or any joint that is ailing. I find that it helps to warm the oil slightly before massaging it into your body.

Taking the Oil Internally

There is a lot of debate when it comes to ingesting essential oils. Many people advise against it because there can be harmful side effects, or you can overdose on the oils if you don't follow the dosages.

In my experience, I have never had an issue taking a couple drops of oil in my tea, but I am always careful of proper dosages. If you are going to use it in your tea, only use a couple of drops, no matter how big your cup of tea is. Only do this once a day.

Sure, there is the tendency to think that if 2 drops is good, then 4 must be better, but that is not the case. Essential oils are highly concentrated, which means the couple drops you are using in your tea is the equivalent to a lot of the fruit or other substance you are using.

Go mild, blend it into the tea you are drinking, and remember that less is more. If you feel sick, dizzy, or like something is off, discontinue ingesting the oils and simply use them topically or diffused into the air. There is evidence to support that you get the same benefits from using these oils topically or through aroma therapy as there is ingesting it.

At the end of the day, you get to decide what you want to do. It's your body, you get to decide. Don't be afraid to try out all three and decide which you want to do for yourself, and have fun with it!

My goal with this book is to give you the freedom you deserve to have with your health, and using essential oils is the best way to do that.

Conclusion

There you have it, everything you need to know to get well versed in the use of essential oils. With this book, you will know not only what kind of oils to use for certain ailments, but you will also know which blends to make and how to administer for the greatest results.

Discover your perfect method, combine that with your favorite blends, and reap the excellent benefits that are sure to follow. In no time at all you will know just what to do with any ailment that arises, no matter what time of the day it is.

I hope this book is able to show you how you can treat any ailment naturally, and you can do it your way. No strict rules, no crazy side effects to worry about, and absolutely none of that medicinal smell that you don't want on you or your children.

Natural remedies are by far the best way to go, and when you know what you are doing, you have the very key you need to make it happen. That is what this book aims to do, and that is exactly what you will be able by the time you have reached this point.

I hope you now feel the confidence I know you should have, and that you are able to treat and prevent a variety of ailments that arise in day to day living. These treatments are the best of the best. They have been around for thousands of years for a reason... they work!

Forget the stress that comes from going to the store and standing in the medication aisle for hours, trying to decide which one is best for you. Now, you can
treat anything you can think of naturally, and naturally you can do it whenever
you please.

Soap Making

Introduction

Research suggests that soap was being used as long ago as 2800 B.C. The ancient Babylonians are thought to have made soap from ashes and fat, although it is unknown as to the extent that soap was used by the general population.

There is also evidence to suggest that the Ancient Egyptians, from approximately 1500 B.C. used a soap product created by mixing fatty animal oils with salt; in effect create a soap which would exfoliate as well! Even the Romans are known to have made a form of soap from urine!

Soap is, in effect a vital part of human history, whether washing blood from your hands in ancient times or destroying microscopic germs; it has always been used. Of course, the more modern versions of soap have been created to leave a pleasant aroma as well as effective and gently washing the skin.

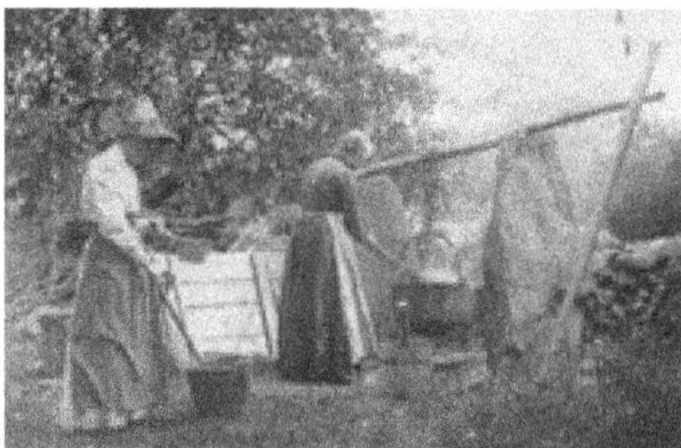

As with most products, soap was originally something that only the richest people could afford; there were very few people capable or licensed to make soap and they guarded their skills carefully. They general used animal oil and parts of plants to create distinctive soaps. This ensured an elite class of customer. However, at the end of the 18th century, a Frenchman discovered a way of chemical making soap; this was the first time soap could be made on a much larger scale. This was the catalyst which drove the price of soap down and made it affordable to a much wider range of people.

This discovery was followed in the early part of the 19th century that soap could be made from glycerin, fats and acid. This made it even cheaper to create soap and is considered to be the foundations of modern soap making; there have been no significant advancements in the science of soap making since. The techniques and principles which were first used approximately two hundred years ago, are still in use today!

Of course, modern technology has changed the understanding of soap, he ingredients are better understood and broken down which has enabled the creation of different types of soap for different situations. Laundry soap is one example of a product which is subtly different to hand soap or even bathing soaps; each has its own role to fulfill. It was only in the 1970's that liquid soap became possible, it has become exceptionally popular since and helps to promote hand washing as well as minimize soap wastage.

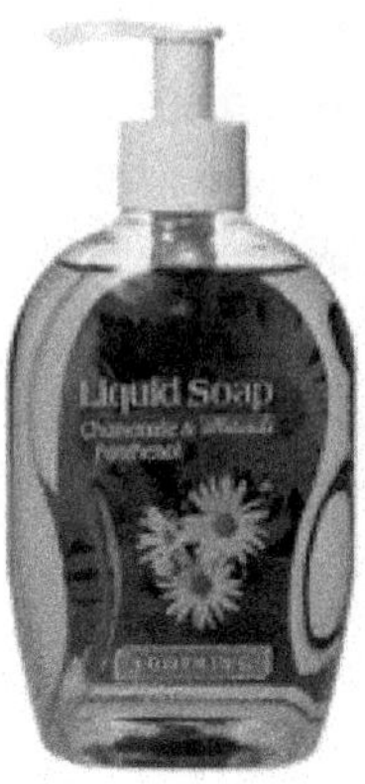

The modern world has a dazzling array if soaps, depending upon your needs, how you wish to smell and even what type of skin you have. These constant changes, improvements and marketing ploys help to keep soap fresh in everyone's mind; a standard bar of soap may be less popular, but the concept and use of soaps has never been so popular. There remains a thriving market for commercially created soaps, there is also a place for those who wish to create their own, homemade soap; a process which I surprisingly easy!

This book will guide you through the best method to make soap and the tools and equipment you will need to complete this task at home. It will also provide you with a selection of twenty five recipes to help you practice and create your own soap; you should then be able to discover and make hundreds of other types of soap!

Chapter 1 – The Need For Soap and How to Make It

In the modern world everyone is aware of the need for soap and its role in helping us to stay clean and healthy, although many people are unaware of how soap works and how regularly it should be used. In fact, there have been many studies into the effects of soap. There are even those who believe that soap is not necessary; the body is able to clean itself. There are two main uses of soap:

Odor Removal

In general research agrees that young children, male or female do not have any odor creating regions. It is, therefore, not necessary for children to use soap in order to remove unpleasant body odors, although soap can still be used to aid them in smelling nice. However, adults, particularly men, do have odor producing regions. Research suggests that it is essential to soap these regions every two days unless you partake in very physical work; in which case every day is essential. Water by itself can significantly reduce the presence if body odor, but will not eliminate it completely. Deodorant will always be needed to assist with reducing and containing odors, the regularity of application will be directly related to the physical duties undertaken. Washing in water will help to reduce body odor but it is more effective when mixed with soap.

Cleanliness

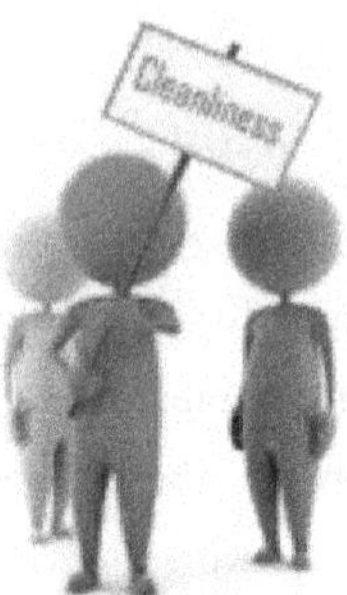

Soap has always been acknowledged as a way to remove dirt and germs from your hands, this is via a process of friction and agitation; in fact, modern soaps have small particles added to them to aid with dirt removal and the removal of excess skin. The abrasive nature of these products will help to leave your skin fresh and glowing and will often help to keep skin conditions at bay. This is because many soap products are becoming more technologically advanced and are able to offer deep pore washes.

There is a school of thought which recommends using only water to clean the skin. However, with the advancements in modern science washing soap can do much more than simple wash your skin, it can help t protect, moisturize and even keep you looking younger for longer.

It is the amount of science behind the soap that often worries people regarding what they are really putting on their face or body. This is one of the main reasons people start to make their own soap; knowing which ingredients have been placed into a bar means you know what you are putting on your body.

The basic process of making any soap is surprisingly simple, in fact, the most important question you will need to ask yourself is whether you wish to handle

Lye yourself or not. Lye is a natural product, also known as Sodium Hydroxide. It is an alkali and can be dangerous; it is capable of making a hole in your fabrics and can burn your skin. However, as long as you handle it with care there will be no issue using it; it is worth noting that you should always use the crystal version of Lye when making salt and it must always be added to the water, not the water to it.

This lye, added in the right quantities to plain water can then be mixed with a variety of different oil. The mixture bonds together to create soap; the main difference between recipes is the additional flavorings and the type of oil used. Every oil has its own specific relationship to lye and must be used in the right quantities.

If the thought of handling lye is to daunting for you at first, then you can purchase a melt and pour soap which is ready to use. As its name suggests, you simply melt it, add your own flavors and pour it into the molds.

The basic tools and equipment required are covered in the next chapter.

Chapter 2 – Tools and Equipment

Thankfully most of the items you will need you will already own; they are normal kitchen utensils. It is worth noting that if you intend to create your own soap on a regular basis is could be worth purchasing equipment specifically for your soap making. This will ensure there is no tang of soap left when cooking your evening meal!

Of course, as well as having all the right tools to hand, you will need to have chosen one of the recipes in this book and made sure that you either have the necessary ingredients or that you have acquired. It can be surprisingly cost effective, as well as fun to make your own soap.

Essential Tools;

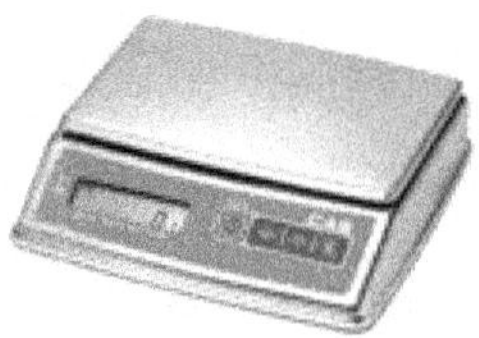

- Scales – the best ones are digital as the more soap you make the more precise you will be regarding the ingredients. This is not just in an effort to reproduce a bar of soap; very small changes in the ingredients can affect the oiliness of the finished product.

- Jars and bowls; these should, ideally, be made of glass.

- Spoons; the best option is to have a wooden one, a metal one and a plastic one.

- Something to contain and shape your soap. You can buy purpose made molds, or you can use a variety of items from your home. Silicon cake tins are one option, but a cardboard box lined with parchment paper can work just as well.

- Gloves are essential as the mixture will be hot, if you decide to use Lye it can also be harmful to your skin. It is also advisable to have some sort of eye protection; this will help prevent splashes from damaging your eyes.

- Vinegar – this will effectively counteract the lye if you do have an accident with it. Having a bottle to hand means you will be ready and able to prevent a disaster!

- A blender; this will make mixing and creating your soap much easier! This should be the handheld, stick type.

- A mixing bowl; the size of this will depend upon the amount of soap you wish to make. For your first attempts it is advisable to make a small amount and get a feel for how to make soap; you will then be able to tweak recipes to suit your own requirements.

- Cloths; you will need to react quickly to any spills; a cloth or paper towel is the best option for this.

You may also wish to consider having a selection of plastic cups handy; this will help you to have the oils and fragrances pre-measured and ready to add to your mix.

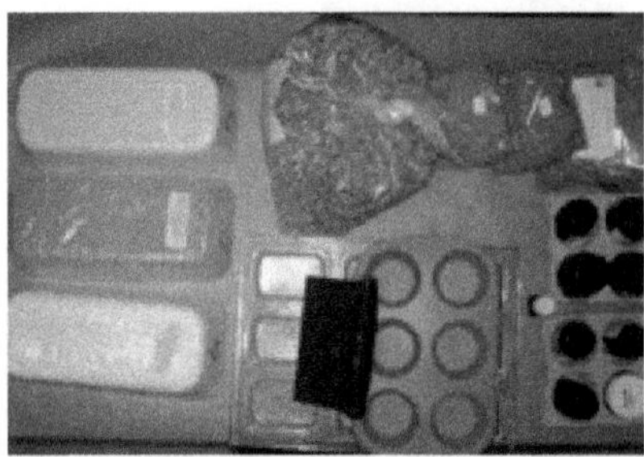

Having got all your tools to hand and your ingredients you will be ready to get started. Perhaps the most important thing to remember when making soap is that preparation is everything. You variety of containers will ensure you are able to measure and prepare all the ingredients before you start mixing them together; doing this will make the process much easier.

Chapter 3 – 10 Fantastic Soaps for All Occasions

There are literally hundreds of potential combinations and types of soap which can be made. In fact, some if the best ones are made as a result of trial and error. The best approach to learning how to make soap is to use the recipes in this book, follow the instructions and understand the process. Once you have mastered this you will be able to change the ingredients and try some of your own combinations, just be sure to note down what you are doing so that you can reproduce it if necessary!

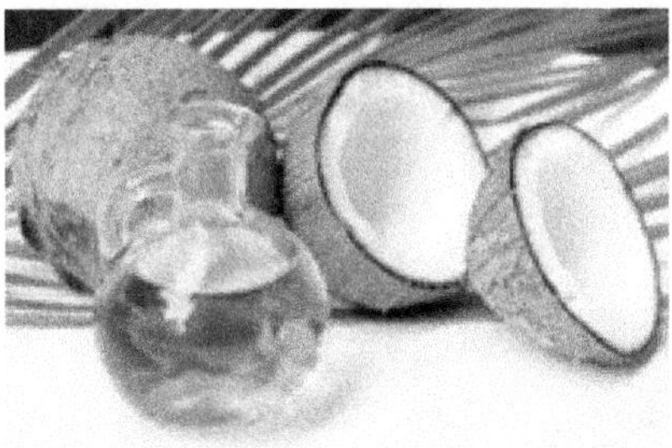

Coconut Oil Soap for Washing

You will need 33 ounces of Coconut Oil, 4.75 ounces of lye and 12.5 ounces of water. If you wish to you can also an a few drops of essential oils.

It is worth noting that there are various types of coconut oil which melt at different temperatures. Ideally you should use one which melts at 76 degrees Fahrenheit, although the recipe will work well with any coconut oil.

The first step is to measure out your three key ingredients. You need to add the water to an empty bowl and then slowly pour the lye into the water. It is advisable to avoid breathing in the fumes whilst doing this. By pouring the lye slowly you will reduced the chance of splash-back and help it to dissolve effectively. The mixture will take approximately ten minutes to go clear.

Separately you will need to put your coconut oil into a pan and heat it to around 120 Fahrenheit. It should melt into a clear liquid.

You can then merge the two liquids carefully together. You can then use your blender to gentle mix it until it appears creamy and light. You can then put the mixture on a low heat and allow to simmer for approximately three quarters of an hour. The soap should be half clear; much like Vaseline. You can check it is ready by making sure it is between seven and ten on a piece of PH paper.

As it cools add your essential oils and then spoon the mixture into your chosen molds. It can cool naturally or cool in the fridge for a quicker result. It is usable straight away although it will be at its best a couple of weeks after production.

Coconut Oil Laundry Soap

This is the same ingredients as the soap for washing but it is important to use one ounce more of lye and half an ounce less of water. The rest of the process is the same but it will make a bar which is more appropriate for washing clothes in.

Olive Oil Soap

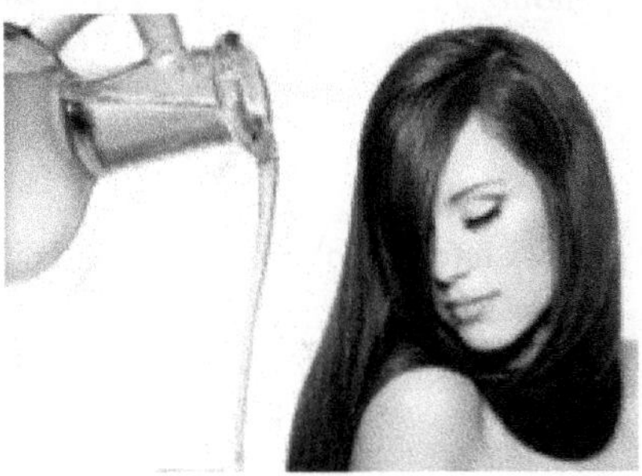

The ingredients in this are very similar to those in coconut oil soap. You will need 50 oz of olive oil, 6.3 oz of Lye and 15 oz of water.

You can choose whether to make the lye first or the olive oil. The water needs to be placed into a good sized bowl or container and the lye slowly added. Again, it will take approximately ten minutes to dissolve completely.

The olive oil will need heating on the stove to ensure it is hot, but not necessarily boiling. You can then slowly add this to the lye mixture and start blending. It should take between five and ten minutes to become nice and creamy.

You will then be able to fill your prepared molds and leave to set. They should, ideally be left overnight and they must be covered to ensure they harden properly.

Poppy seed Soap

Instead of using lye it is possible to use a soap base. This can be bought at most craft shops and will vary in price depending upon what the base is created from.

You will also need poppy seeds and you may wish to use coloring to ensure you soap look good.

Ideally you should use 10 oz of your soap base. Cut it into small pieces and place in a jug or bowl. This can then be melted in the microwave. Once melted add a teaspoon of poppy seeds and a few drops of coloring if required. You can also add a fragrance if desired. Mix all the ingredients and pour into your mold.

Put the mold in the fridge for fifteen minutes and then the soap is ready to us.

Jasmine and Rosewood

You will need one teaspoon of kaolin clay, two teaspoons of titanium dioxide, half an ounce of jasmine and half an ounce of rosewood. You will also need five ounces of lye, twelve ounce of water and possibly yellow oxide.

Start by adding the lye slowly to the water and leaving it to clear, (as before). Then mix the titanium dioxide and clay together; you will need to grind them to ensure there are no lumps. You can then add the jasmine, rosewood and titanium mixture to the lye, stirring carefully whilst doing so. You may also wish to add a little yellow oxide to improve the color of the soap.

Once mixed, you can pour into your chosen molds and leave for twenty four hours before cutting into blocks. It is best to leave the cut soap for three weeks before using it.

Calendula soap

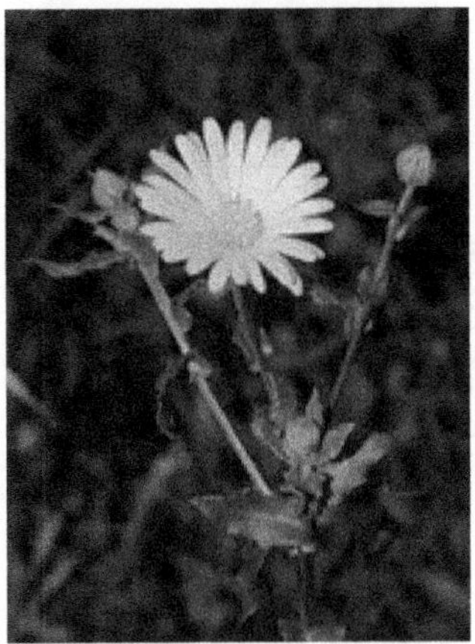

You will need; 21 ounces of olive oil, 14 ounces of coconut oil, 2 ounces of castor oil, 5 ounces of sunflower oil, 13 ounces of calendula tea, 6 ounces of lye and 13 ounces of water.

As usual measure out the water and slowly add the lye to it, then wait for it to become clear. Mix the oils together and heat them until they nearly reach boiling point, the slowly add them to the lye mix. Now simply add the calendula tea and blend until creamy.

You will then be able to pour them into your molds and use your soap in a couple of weeks.

Shampoo bar

As its name suggests this product is perfect for washing your hair! You will need; 9 ounces of olive oil and coconut oil, 4 ounces of coconut oil and of jojoba oil, two ounces of shea butter and cocoa butter, one ounce beeswax, four ounces water and four ounces of lye,

As usual, slowly add the lye to the water. Whilst this is becoming clear, mix all the oils and the beeswax together. This mixture can then be heated, but not brought to the boil. Now mix the lye with the oils and b lend until it is thick and creamy. The mixture should then be allowed to simmer for one hour and then you can pour it into its molds. After twenty four hours the mold can be cut into bar and left to cool further; although they can be used straight away.

Gin and Tonic Soap

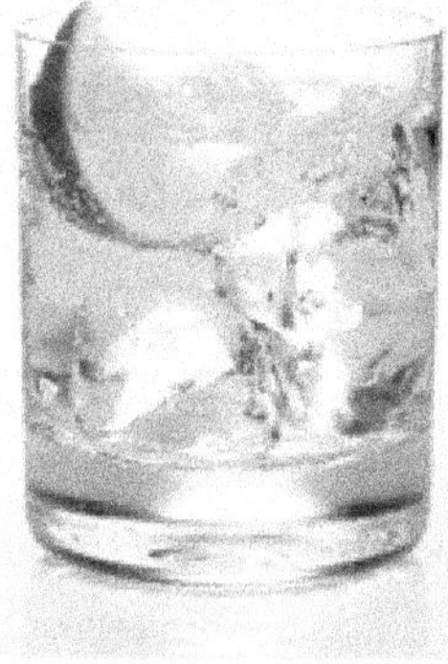

As with all the recipes you will need to pour 5 ounces of lye into 12 ounces of water and allow it to mix to makes its own, clear liquid.

You will then need to heat 3.5 ounces of olive oil, 2.5 ounces coconut oil, 1.5 ounces shea butter, 1.5 ounces lard and 1 ounce of castor oil. Do not allow it to boil before you add it the lye and water. This should then be left for approximately six hours; then add half an ounce of juniper oil, 3 ounces of lemon essential oil and a teaspoon of kaolin clay. Cut after twenty four hours and use after three weeks.

Lanolin Shaving soap

Lanolin is a natural moisturizer and is perfect for shaving with as it prevents the skin from drying out as you shave. To create it you will need the following ingredients:

1 ounce kokum butter, 2 ounces lanolin, 2 ounces of shea butter, 11 ounces of coconut oil, 10 ounces of rice bran oil, 7 ounces palm kernel flakes, 1 ounce pumpkin oil. You will also need 5 ounces of lye and twelve ounces of water and you can add any essential oil you like to create a pleasant fragrance.

Mix the water and lye as usual, whilst waiting for it to cool and clear you should mix all the other oils and butter together, heat all these ingredients until they are all melted. Ideally you should merge the two liquids at approximately 110 degrees. Just prior to merging you can add the essential oils.

Once merged blend into a cream and then put into your molds. Keep them wrapped and insulated for twenty four hours before cutting them to size. Then keep them stored for another three weeks before using them.

Aloe Vera Soap

As with all these soaps you will need to prepare a mixture of lye and water before mixing the oils whilst heating and then combining the two mixtures. For this recipe you need 10 ounces of lye and 7 ounces of lye.

The oils which need to be mixed are 15 ounces Coconut oil, 13 Ounces olive oil and 10 ounces lard. Just prior to mixing them with the lye, it is essential to add the aloe gel. Once they have been blended it will take about 48 hours for them to be set enough to cut and a further four weeks before they should be used.

Chapter 4 – 10 Food Flavoured Soap

There are a great many number of soaps which have been created using food flavorings; this can add a beautiful fragrance to any soap and can also provide a host of health benefits. The following recipes all use the same approach as the soaps already described. Every soap mixture requires 12 ounces of water and 5 ounces of lye. Your soap making should start by carefully mixing these together. The mixture will go cloudy and become extremely hot. Whilst this is settling you should mix the oils and warm them. Add any essential oils can be added prior to mixing lye and the oils.

The following recipes all adopt this approach, as such, only the ingredients and items which need to be noted will appear:

Honey Soap

Additional ingredients to the lye and water are; one tablespoon of buttermilk fragrance oil, half a tablespoon of vanilla flavoring, orange color, (you can choose not to use this) and 3 ounces of honey. Your choice of honey will affect the color of your soap and hence affect whether you wish to use the orange coloring or not. You may also like to find bee molds or honeycombs to make the soap more fun!

Chai Latte Soap

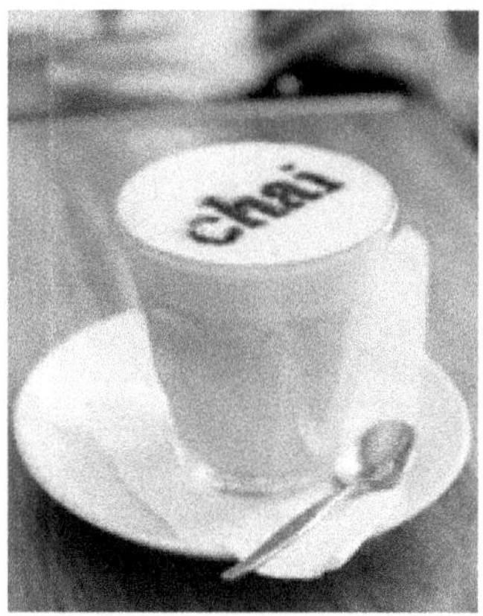

You will need five ounces of coconut oil, five ounces of olive oil and five ounces of olive oil. You will then also need two ounces of cocoa butter and two ounces of castor oil. The ingredients should all be mixed and blended as per the usual instructions. However, you will notice it thickens quickly when blended. It can also look fantastic to make them in plastic cups; you can even decorate the top and make two batches to create the milky layer and the coffee layer; so that they look like a coffee/ latte!

Chocolate Soap

Who wouldn't want to wash in a bar of chocolate! This soap is created to look exactly like a bar of chocolate, or, if stood on its end it could be a hot chocolate!

You will need; four ounces of olive oil, two and a half ounces of coconut oil, two ounces of lard, one ounce of avocado oil and half an ounce of castor oil. You will also need two teaspoons of whole milk powder, two of coffee granules, one teaspoon of cocoa powder and 2 teaspoons of vanilla flecks. Additionally, you will need two teaspoons of red clay and two of brown clay, along with two teaspoons of vanilla flavoring.

The oils should be mixed with the lye as usual; once it has been blended and become creamy you can add the extra ingredients and pour into a mold. As usual the soap can be cut to size within twenty four hours and then left for three weeks to harden

Candy cane Christmas Soap

You will need; 4 ounces of olive oil, 2.5 ounces of coconut oil, 2 ounces of lard, 1 ounce of avocado oil and half an ounce of castor oil. You will also need two teaspoons of peppermint essence, one teaspoon of vanilla essence, one table-spoon kaolin clay, half a teaspoon of red oxide and half a teaspoon of green oxide.

Mix the lye and heat the oils as normal. Then add the vanilla and peppermint essence and blend in the kaolin clay. Now split the soap mix into three bowls. Add the red oxide to one bowl and the green oxide to another. Now alternate and swirl the colors separately into the molds. They should create a candy cane effect. As usual leave for twenty four hours before cutting and leave for a further thre weeks before using.

Milk Soap

You will need 20 ounces of milk, twenty ounces of coconut oil, four ounces of your preferred fragrance and four pounds of lard. As usual you can start by preparing the lye and water. You will need to wait for approximately an hour for the mixture to lower its temperature to approximately eighty degrees. You can then add the cold milk. Whilst the temperature is settling again you can prepare the oil and the lard; merging them and heating them to ninety degrees. You can then add the oils to the lye and keep stirring until it is thick.

You can then pour it into your chosen molds, but you must cover the mold with plastic and a blanket; this will ensure the heat is retained which will effectively cook the soap. Again, after twenty four hours it can be cut into shapes or the size required. It should be allowed to air dry for another four weeks before being used.

Creamy Orange Soap

This soap requires two tablespoons of annatto seeds, two ounces of olive oil, two tablespoons of poppy seeds, one ounce of essential oil; orange flavored preferably and one and a half ounces of peppermint oil.

Mix the oils heat them with the essential oils and seeds. The simply merge them with the lye mixture and blend. You should then be able to pour the mixture into the mold and leave for twenty four hours to set.

The seeds will act as an exfoliate in the soap making it very good at restoring dry skin.

Marbled Beer Soap

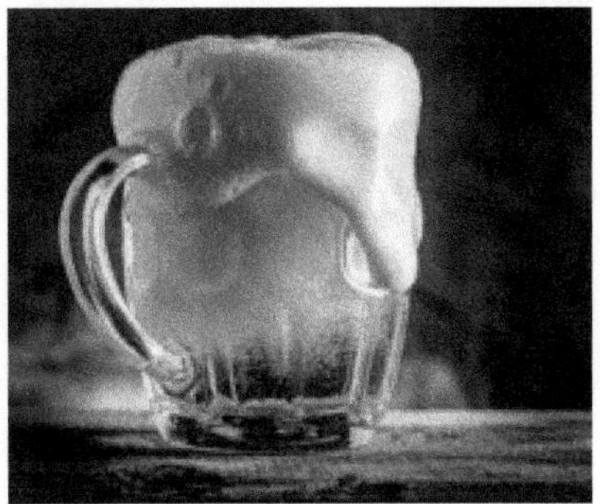

You may not know whether to wash with this or drink it, but it will certainly make a good talking point and a gift. You need four and a half ounces of chilled beer, five ounces of palm kernel oil, three and a half ounces of palm oil and the same of coconut oil. You will also need one ounce of Babassu oil, five ounces of rapeseed oil, five ounces of sunflower oil, one ounce of castor oil, two ounces of soybean oil and half an ounce of cedar wood essential oil.

Having collected all the ingredients together you should introduce half of the lye to the water as normal; the other half should be poured into the cold beer. Heat your oils and merge them with your water and with your beer; roughly half the oils inn each pot. You will not be able to blend this to a thick consistency. Now pour the two mixtures into the mold, you can alternate or even pour at the same time to achieve a marble effect. You can then cover it for between twenty four and forty eight hours, keeping it warm to help it set.

Apple Cider Soap

In this mixture, instead of adding your lye to water, add it to nine ounces of chilled cider. You can then mix your oils; 15 ounces of olive oil, 2 ounces castor oil, 8 ounces coconut oil, 2 ounces cocoa butter and 3 ounces of avocado oil. You can also add a touch of ginger or cinnamon, to your own preference.

Cinnamon Soap

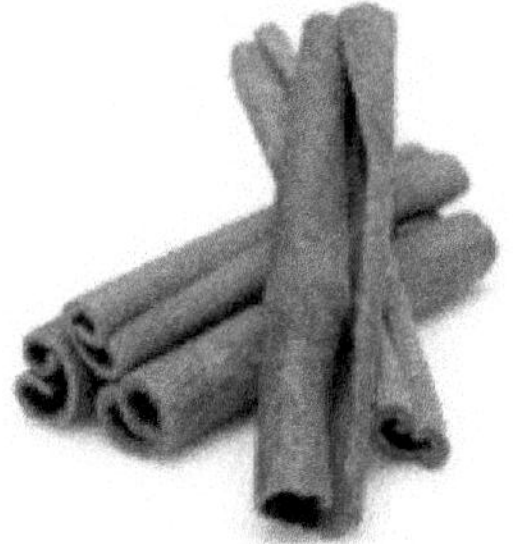

The oil mixture consists of 3.5 ounces olive oil, 2.5 ounces coconut oil, 1.5 ounces lard, 1.5 ounces shea butter and 1 ounce castor oil. You will also need a teaspoon of ground cinnamon, a tablespoon of white clay and two teaspoons of cinnamon essential oil. The essential oil, ground cinnamon and clay should be added at the end of the process; just before you pour the soap into the molds.

Tea Tree Soap

This soap requires an oil mixture of 14 ounces olive oil, 10 ounces coconut oil, 4 ounces sweet almond oil, 4 ounces avocado oil and two teaspoons of tea tree essential oil. Again, the tea tree essential oil should be added just before the soap is poured into the mold. After twenty four hours you can cut the mold and it can be left to air dry for up to six weeks.

Chapter 5 – A selection of fun Soaps – 5 Recipes

The list of soaps you can make is endless; in fact, you are only limited by your imagination. It is even possible to use a   soap base instead of the lye to avoid the danger involved in dealing with lye. The following five recipes are done using a soap base but are all worth trying: Each recipe requires you to melt the soap base in the microwave and then add the necessary ingredients to make your soap. Solid particles will go to the bottom of the soap unless you allow it to set a little first. The soap can set in as little as three hours although it is always recommended to chill it overnight.

Herbs & Citrus Soap

Simply put some soap base in a bowl, or grate an old bar of soap and warm it up. Soap base can be warmed in the microwave whereas old soap is best to do on the stove. Simply choose your favorite hers, such as mint or rosemary and grind or puree them into tiny pieces. Once your base has melted, and them to it and stir in. Pour the soap into the molds and leave to cool for an hour; you can speed the cooling and setting process by putting them in the freezer.

Mocha Soap

Simply melt the soap base and add approximately one tablespoon of coffee and cocoa powder to it. This will create a fantastic smelling soap. To help create the mocha effect you could melt a second soap base and add a little white colorant to help create the milky mocha effect. To make a stunning display pour the two soap bases into a cup at the same time; sprinkle with chocolate powder and you will have a soap which looks like a mocha!

Honey & Dandelion Soap

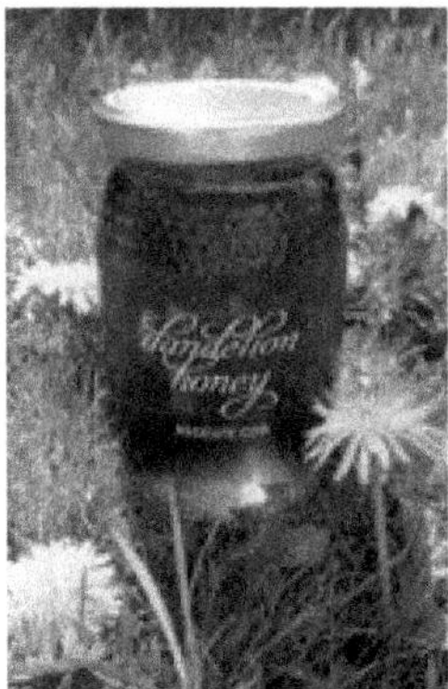

You can use dandelions to make your soap but this may result in bits in your soap! It is better to make a dandelion tea and use this to flavor the soap. The ingredients you will need are are; 10 ounces of dandelion tea and one ounce of honey. These two ingredients need to be added base soap once you have melted it. You should keep the soap simmering to ensure the honey and dandelion tea has mixed completely.

Again, this soap should be set within a few hours; ideally it should be used within three months of its first use.

Cucumber soap

Cucumber is known to clean and refresh any skin, adding it to a soap means you have access to it whenever you need a boost.

To make the soap you will need the pulp of one cucumber. The best way of doing this is to peel and grate it into the smallest pieces possible. Again, you will need to add this to the soap base and warm the entire mixture. It should be set within a few hours.

Soap on a stick

This can be a great way to introduce children to soap and remind everyone of how important it is to wash. Putting soap on a stick may make it appear like a lollipop; you will need to be careful that your children do not try to eat them!

You will need lollipop sticks; clear glycerin, food coloring and fragrance oil. Simply start by cutting the glycerin into blocks and putting them in a bowl before melting them in the microwave. You can then stir in your fragrance, the food coloring and any specific flavor your children may want to wash in. The mixture can then be poured into a mold and a lollipop stick attached. To get the soap to set it is best to put the molds in the freezer for ten minutes.

Conclusion

Making soap is cost effective, fun and will allow you to be extremely creative. There are literally hundreds of recipes, some will use lye whilst others use old soaps or soap base. It can often be good to start with the soap bases and move up to using lye mixtures. This will ensure you are comfortable with all the processes and measuring before tackling the more dangerous approach.

Providing you adopt a cautious approach to lye and always have a bottle of vinegar on standby you will be perfectly safe and capable of using lye. It does give off noxious fumes when first mixed, if possible it is better to mix it outside. However, providing you adopt the right approach you will not have an issue using this product.

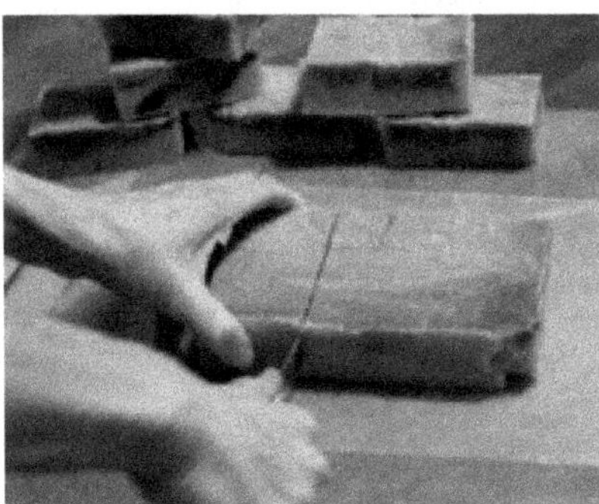

It is also fascinating to note how the scent and even the feel of soap can be completely changed just by increasing or decreasing the quantities of the ingredients. There is no reason why you cannot adjust the quantities or even add extra items to any recipe to make your own variant of soap; at the worst it will not work properly and you can simply start again!

Making your own soap is becoming increasingly popular; this is not just because it is much cheaper than buying luxury soap; there is also a sense of satisfaction and achievement when you make your first batch. In fact, it is so easy to get started in that there is really no excuse for anyone not to have a go!

20 Natural Homemade Soap Recipes With Easy Instructions

Introduction

There you are, in the department store once more, reading over all of the soap labels, trying to find that one soap that is perfect for you. You want a soap that is right for your skin type, smells like you want it to smell, and something that you are able to modify for any reason you want.

But, most importantly, you want a soap that is all natural. You know how harmful chemicals can be, and that avoiding these chemicals is the best thing to do for your health, your cleanliness, and most of all, your happiness.

"But I don't want to spend twenty dollars on a bar of soap."

"I know what I want, but I don't want to use lye or expose my younger children to the harmful substance."

"I have always wanted to make soap, but I hear that there is a lot involved, and it sounds hard. I don't know if I would be able to do it."

It's true, if you have never made your own soap before, you are sure to run into some initial roadblocks. Whether you are told a number of facts that people offer, you are scared off by all the warnings that you read on directions, or if you simply don't want to have to purchase all of the special equipment.

There has to be a better way, and there has to be a more family friendly alternative to the classic way of making soap. Thankfully, there is. And this is the book that is going to show you how to make that happen. Using all natural ingredients, and combining both fun and safety, this book is going to show you exactly how you can make the soap that you want quickly and easily.

Roll up your sleeves and get ready for the fast and fun way to make soap, and say goodbye to all the hassle you have dealt with in the past. Soap making has never been better, safer, or easier.

Unlock the secret to making your own soap in the safest way possible, and get ready to embrace a new hobby that is going to last a lifetime. No more mess, no more stress, and no more worry. This is your perfect guide to making all natural soap.

What are you waiting for?

Jump on in.

Chapter 1 – Getting Started: Making Soap Your Way

No doubt if you have ever attempted to make your own soap, or if you have ever researched making your own soap, you were met with the fact that you have to use lye.

While in and of itself lye isn't dangerous, there are a lot of other factors that come into play that makes it something you don't want to have around your children if you can help it. Of course, people have been making soap with lye for thousands of years, but why have to worry about something when you don't have to, right?

With the soaps you will find with this book, you are going to have the perfect opportunity to make your own soaps, and never have to deal with lye yourself. Some of the ingredients you will use to make your soaps may contain lye, but I wanted to provide a book that allowed you to make soap your way without having to deal with any lye directly.

The best way to avoid having to handle lye directly, is to use a base soap.

Now, when it comes to the world of 'base soaps', you will find that there are hundreds of different options for you to choose from. You can find some that are practically ready to go as is, or you can find the most basic of the basic and add anything and everything you want to them.

The biggest plus to using a base soap is that the lye is going to be found in here, and you won't have to worry about having to deal with it directly. You can find bars of soap, liquid soaps, and virtually anything in between, just take a look on Amazon if you aren't sure where to find them locally.

If you want the fastest and easiest method of making your own soap, purchase a soap at the grocery store that is as plain as can be. You can modify this as much as you please, turning it into the soap that you want.

When I am in a real pinch, and I want soap right now, I will go to the store and purchase a white bar of soap with no additives. I take this home and use it as my soap base, and the result is exactly the soap I want how I want it.

Of course, as with anything you try for the first time, you will need to go through some practice, trial, and error before you get just what you are after, but the more you stick with it, the easier it is going to become.

My biggest piece of advice to anyone that is starting to make soap for themselves is to have fun with it, and be willing to laugh at the results.

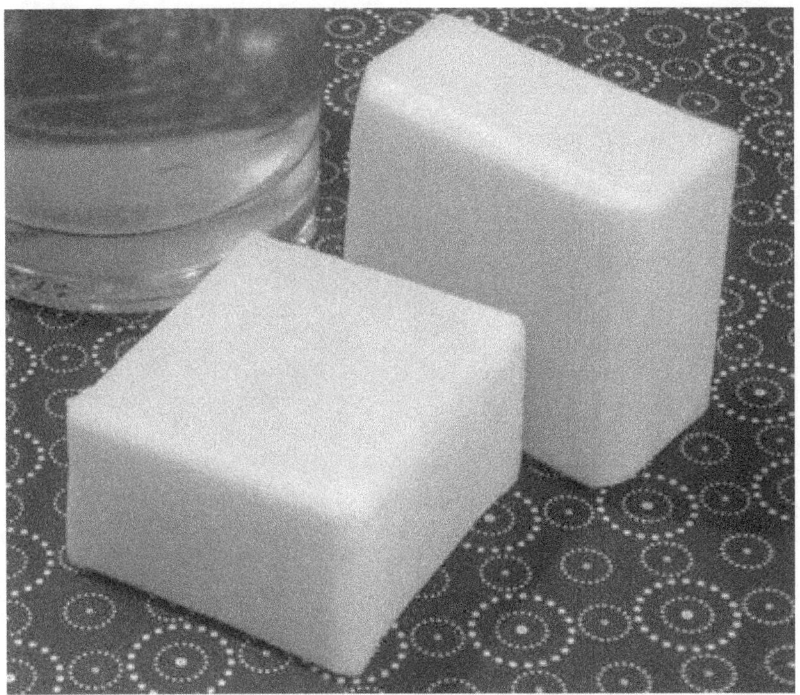

At the end of the day, the soap you make is going to clean you, but you may not get the look or scent that you are after when you started. This is where you need to practice and stick with it.

The more you do, the more experience you will have, and the better your soap is going to turn out, no matter how much or how little time you have.

One of the major drawbacks to making soap the old fashioned way is how long it takes for the soap to set up. With this method of making your own soap, you don't have to worry about tons of time involved, and you will be able to modify how you please.

The other ingredients you need are simple, whether they are essential oils, herbs, dried flowers, or things like that. You can even add glitter or other charm to your soap… personalize it as much as you like!

Chapter 2 – Easy Custom Molded Soaps

One of the most fun things you can do with your own homemade soap is mold it to look like whatever you like.

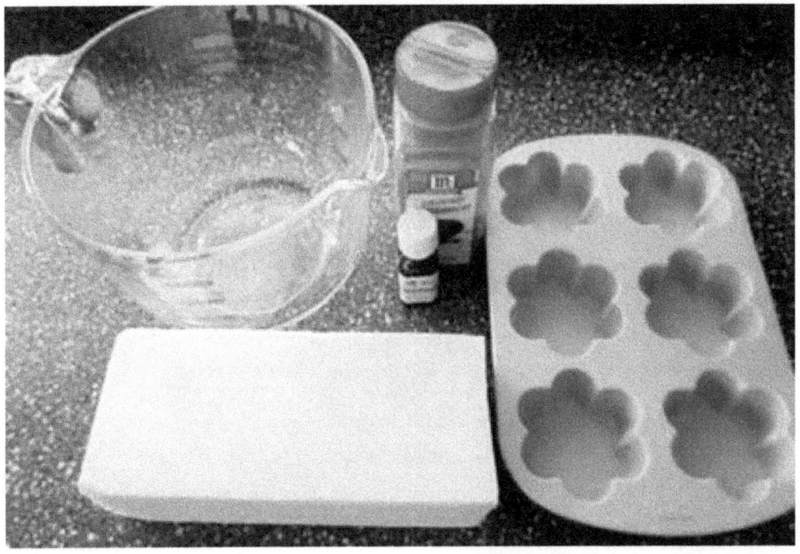

Use these soaps directly in your hands, or use them with a loofa or a washcloth. They will lather as much as you want them to, but you may have to work them a little with the wash cloth to get them really foamy.

If you want them to lather more, use more of the base soap in the recipe. Each recipe calls for a single bar of the base soap, but if you increase the base soap by another half bar, you will get a much foamier soap at the end.

You can do this by hand, or you can pour the hot, melted soap into molds and let it harden that way. Get creative with it and try out anything... there's no wrong way to do it.

Insider's Tip:

I have used cookie cutters to get the basic shape for some of my soaps. If you want to have the same size and shape of soaps, this is a great way to go about that.

If the bars get too hard for you to use your cookie cutter, you can always re-melt them and use the cookie cutter over. Have fun and try a variety of shapes and sizes... there's no end to the possibilities of what you may come up with!

The Little Heartthrob Soap

What you will need:

All natural base soap

1 teaspoon beat juice

12 drops rose essential oil

Small handful dried rose petals

Directions:

Cut your base soap into smaller pieces, and melt with 1 teaspoon coconut oil in a pan on the stove. Stir often, until it is completely melted.

Add in the essential oils slowly, stirring the entire time. Remove from heat and set on a hot pad.

Keep an eye on the soap, and once it begins to harden, stir in any extra additive you wish to add. Let harden more, and once it is cool enough for you to handle it, form into the shape you desire.

Let sit for 24 hours, and your soap is done!

Luscious Lavender Balls

What you will need:

All natural base soap

Lemon zest

6 drops lemon oil

12 drops lavender essential oil

Handful dried purple flower petals

Directions:

Cut your base soap into smaller pieces, and melt with 1 teaspoon coconut oil in a pan on the stove. Stir often, until it is completely melted.

Add in the essential oils slowly, stirring the entire time. Remove from heat and set on a hot pad.

Keep an eye on the soap, and once it begins to harden, stir in any extra additive you wish to add. Let harden more, and once it is cool enough for you to handle it, form into the shape you desire.

Let sit for 24 hours, and your soap is done!

Happy Wash

What you will need:

All natural base soap

12 drops bubblegum aroma essential oil

9 drops beet juice (you want your soap to end up a light pink color, so add as much or as little as you like to get the color you want)

2 tablespoons Epsom salt (for exfoliation, add as much or as little as you like)

Directions:

Cut your base soap into smaller pieces, and melt with 1 teaspoon coconut oil in a pan on the stove. Stir often, until it is completely melted.

Add in the essential oils slowly, stirring the entire time. Remove from heat and set on a hot pad.

Keep an eye on the soap, and once it begins to harden, stir in any extra additive you wish to add. Let harden more, and once it is cool enough for you to handle it, form into the shape you desire.

Let sit for 24 hours, and your soap is done!

Snowballs

What you will need:

1 base bar

18 drops peppermint oil

1 teaspoon glitter

Directions:

Cut your base soap into smaller pieces, and melt with 1 teaspoon coconut oil in a pan on the stove. Stir often, until it is completely melted.

Add in the essential oils slowly, stirring the entire time. Remove from heat and set on a hot pad.

Keep an eye on the soap, and once it begins to harden, stir in any extra additive you wish to add. Let harden more, and once it is cool enough for you to handle it, form into the shape you desire.

Let sit for 24 hours, and your soap is done!

Apples to Oranges

What you will need:

1 bar base soap

12 drops orange oil

¼ cup crushed, dried orange peel

Directions:

Cut your base soap into smaller pieces, and melt with 1 teaspoon coconut oil in a pan on the stove. Stir often, until it is completely melted.

Add in the essential oils slowly, stirring the entire time. Remove from heat and set on a hot pad.

Keep an eye on the soap, and once it begins to harden, stir in any extra additive you wish to add. Let harden more, and once it is cool enough for you to handle it, form into the shape you desire.

Let sit for 24 hours, and your soap is done!

Chapter 3 – Satisfying Hand Soaps

There are few things that can compare to a sweet and lathery hand soap when you need to freshen up. That is exactly what these soaps are meant to do, and it is exactly what they accomplish.

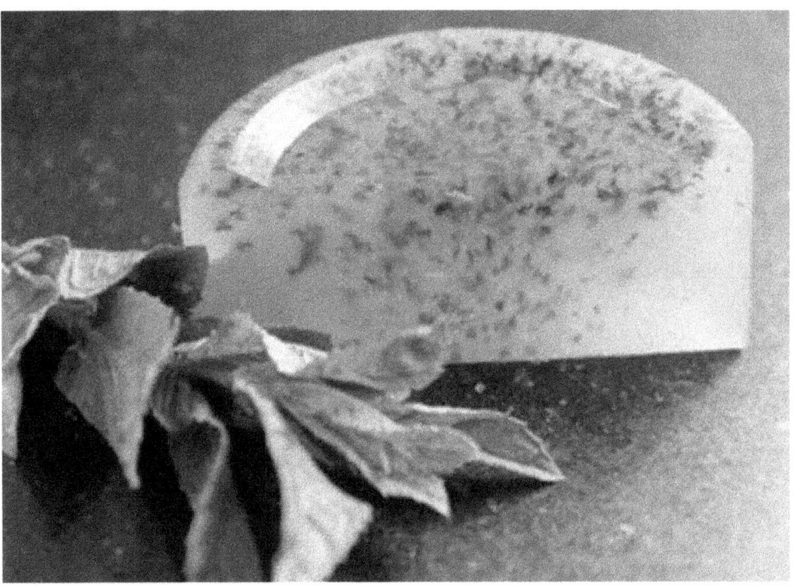

Your hands get dirtier than any other part of you in a day, and when you are getting ready to go from one activity to another, you need something that is going to get the job done quickly and leave you feeling refreshed. These hand soaps are going to do that very thing, taking out all of the hassle out of washing your hands.

They won't dry out your skin, they don't leave a residue, and they won't take long to use. You can make a bottle to put next to every sink in your house.

Make up several bottles and you will never have to worry about what to keep beside your sinks again.

The Quickie

What you will need:

1 bottle clear, all natural unscented hand soap

12 drops apple essential fragrance oil

5 drops lime essential oil

1 glass soap dispenser

Directions:

Pour your liquid soap into a glass bowl, and stir in the essential oils.

If you choose to add in any other extra, make sure they are very small… small enough to fit through the pump of the soap dispenser.

Stir these in, and add 1 to 2 teaspoons of water to achieve the desired consistency.

Pour into your soap dispenser, and you are set!

Liquid Silk

What you will need:

1 bottle clear unscented, all natural hand soap

12 drops lavender essential oil

10 drops lilac essential oil

4 drops hibiscus aroma therapy oil

1 teaspoon water

1 glass jar soap dispenser

Directions:

Pour your liquid soap into a glass bowl, and stir in the essential oils.

If you choose to add in any other extra, make sure they are very small... small enough to fit through the pump of the soap dispenser.

Stir these in, and add 1 to 2 teaspoons of water to achieve the desired consistency.

Pour into your soap dispenser, and you are set!

Princess Wash

What you will need:

1 bottle liquid, all natural, unscented hand soap

1 teaspoon golden glitter

1 teaspoon chunky glitter

10 drops sunflower essential oil

1 tablespoon water

1 glass jar soap dispenser

Directions:

Pour your liquid soap into a glass bowl, and stir in the essential oils.

If you choose to add in any other extra, make sure they are very small... small enough to fit through the pump of the soap dispenser.

Stir these in, and add 1 to 2 teaspoons of water to achieve the desired consistency.

Pour into your soap dispenser, and you are set!

Moisture Matters Hand Soap

What you will need:

1 bottle all natural, unscented liquid hand soap

1 tablespoon fractionated coconut oil

¼ cup water

20 drops peppermint essential oil

Directions:

Pour your liquid soap into a glass bowl, and stir in the essential oils.

If you choose to add in any other extra, make sure they are very small... small enough to fit through the pump of the soap dispenser.

Stir these in, and add 1 to 2 teaspoons of water to achieve the desired consistency.

Pour into your soap dispenser, and you are set!

The Bacteria Buster

What you will need:

1 bottle unscented, all natural, clear liquid hand soap

1 glass jar soap dispenser

¼ cup water

15 drops tea tree oil

5 drops garlic

10 drops orange essential oil

Directions:

Pour your liquid soap into a glass bowl, and stir in the essential oils.

If you choose to add in any other extra, make sure they are very small… small enough to fit through the pump of the soap dispenser.

Stir these in, and add 1 to 2 teaspoons of water to achieve the desired consistency.

Pour into your soap dispenser, and you are set!

Chapter 4 – Head And Shoulders, Knees And Toes: Body Wash

As with the other bases you find on Amazon, you will find liquids along with the bars. If you want to make body wash, I recommend you use a liquid base rather than using hand soap to get the liquid effect.

You can always use a bar soap for a body wash, but I find you just can't beat the luxury of a silky smooth body wash. You will find that this chapter is all about the liquids, but if you want to try out the same recipes and use a bar instead, go for it!

The more you explore, the more you are going to discover new and exciting ways to make soaps you and your family will love.

Use these soaps directly in your hands, or use them with a loofa or a washcloth. They will lather as much as you want them to, but you may have to work them a little with the wash cloth to get them really foamy.

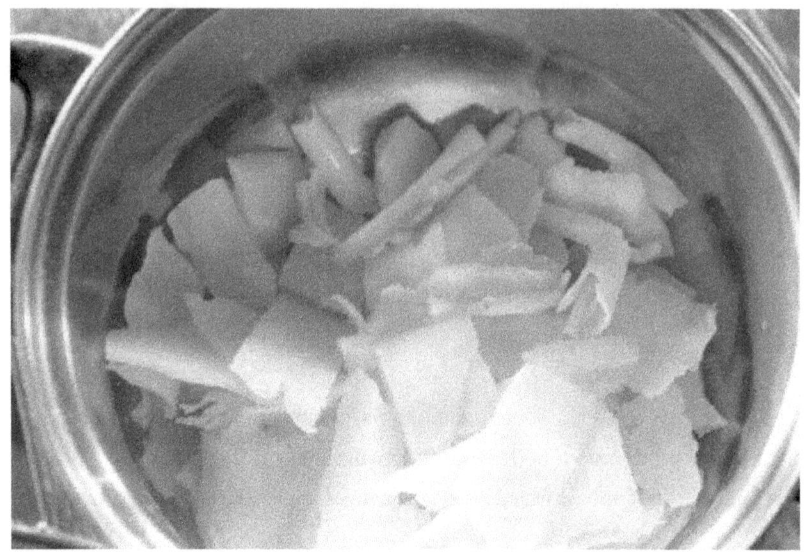

https://www.google.com/search?
q=home+made+soap+no+lye&espv=2&biw=1366&bih=667&source=lnms&tbm=isch&sa=X&ved=0ahUKEwidl5H-
Fo4POAhVM7GMKHQpJCGkQ_AUICCgD#imgrc=_

If you want them to lather more, use more of the base soap in the recipe. Each recipe calls for a single bar of the base soap, but if you increase the base soap by another half bar, you will get a much foamier soap at the end.

You will end up with a better blended product, and you will be able to keep it fresher, longer. Look around on Amazon, or anywhere else you get your base soaps, and find the perfect liquid base for your body wash.

The Spa Spoiler

What you will need:

1 bottle liquid base soap

15 drops rose essential oil

15 drops hibiscus aroma therapy oil

1 tablespoon fractionated coconut oil

Jar with pump for storage and use

Directions:

Pour the liquid base soap in a bowl.

Add in the essential oils, and the two tablespoons of water.

Break up the extra additions you are adding into your soap. You want body wash to be more a liquid than a solid, so the smaller the better with the extras.

Stir everything together, and pour into your dispenser.

That's it! Your new body wash is ready to spoil you whenever you are ready!

Red Velvet Deluxe Body Wash

What you will need:

15 drops beet juice

1 bottle liquid base soap (all natural)

1 tablespoon dark chocolate powder

15 drops vanilla essential oil

Jar with pump for storage and use

Directions:

Pour the liquid base soap in a bowl.

Add in the essential oils, and the two tablespoons of water.

Break up the extra additions you are adding into your soap. You want body wash to be more a liquid than a solid, so the smaller the better with the extras.

Stir everything together, and pour into your dispenser.

That's it! Your new body wash is ready to spoil you whenever you are ready!

Catch Me If You Can Body Wash

What you will need:

1 bottle all natural liquid base soap

15 drops sandalwood essential oil

5 drops tea tree essential oil

2 tablespoons water

Jar with pump for storage and use

Directions:

Pour the liquid base soap in a bowl.

Add in the essential oils, and the two tablespoons of water.

Break up the extra additions you are adding into your soap. You want body wash to be more a liquid than a solid, so the smaller the better with the extras.

Stir everything together, and pour into your dispenser.

That's it! Your new body wash is ready to spoil you whenever you are ready!

The Birds And The Bees Body Wash

What you will need:

1 bottle all natural base soap, liquid

12 drops spring rain aroma therapy essential oil

5 drops hibiscus essential oil

5 drops rose essential oil

2 tablespoons water

Jar with pump for storage and use

Directions:

Pour the liquid base soap in a bowl.

Add in the essential oils, and the two tablespoons of water.

Break up the extra additions you are adding into your soap. You want body wash to be more a liquid than a solid, so the smaller the better with the extras.

Stir everything together, and pour into your dispenser.

That's it! Your new body wash is ready to spoil you whenever you are ready!

Cash On The Barrel Body Wash

What you will need:

1 bottle all natural liquid base soap

Glass jar with pump for storage and use

2 tablespoons water

15 drops tea tree oil

10 drops orange oil

5 drops lemon essential oil

Directions:

Pour the liquid base soap in a bowl.

Add in the essential oils, and the two tablespoons of water.

Break up the extra additions you are adding into your soap. You want body wash to be more a liquid than a solid, so the smaller the better with the extras.

Stir everything together, and pour into your dispenser.

That's it! Your new body wash is ready to spoil you whenever you are ready!

Chapter 5 – Something For Everyone Soaps

There are always specialty soaps on your wish list. If you give it any thought, you know that it doesn't take you long to think of the perfect soap you wish you could have, or the perfect soap you wish you could make for yourself.

That is what this chapter is about. The special soaps that you want to keep on hand for those nights when you want that bit of extra pampering. Whether you want a soap that is going to erase wrinkles, you want a soap that is going to get rid of acne, or you just want that extra kiss of moisture, you are going to get just what you are after with this selection.

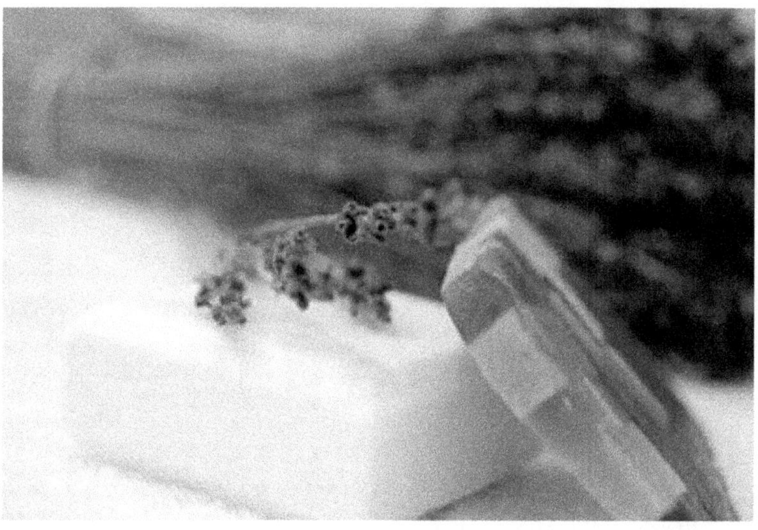

Use these soaps directly in your hands, or use them with a loofa or a washcloth. They will lather as much as you want them to, but you may have to work them a little with the wash cloth to get them really foamy.

If you want them to lather more, use more of the base soap in the recipe. Each recipe calls for a single bar of the base soap, but if you increase the base soap by another half bar, you will get a much foamier soap at the end.

Make up a wide selection for yourself, then make up a few gift baskets to keep on hand for when you are invited to your next get together. There's no way you can go wrong when you bring all natural to the table!

The Wrinkle Eraser

What you will need:

1 bar base soap, all natural and free of any additives

10 drops myrrh essential oil

5 drops frankincense essential oil

5 drops patchouli essential oil

2 teaspoons coconut oil (divided. Use 1 in the mixture and melt with another)

Directions:

Cut your base soap into smaller pieces, and melt with 1 teaspoon coconut oil in a pan on the stove. Stir often, until it is completely melted.

Add in the essential oils slowly, stirring the entire time. Remove from heat and set on a hot pad.

Keep an eye on the soap, and once it begins to harden, stir in any extra additive you wish to add. Let harden more, and once it is cool enough for you to handle it, form into the shape you desire.

Let sit for 24 hours, and your soap is done!

The Acne Blaster Face Soap

What you will need:

1 bar base soap, make sure it is all natural and free of any kind of additives

15 drops tea tree oil

10 drops ginger oil

5 drops cinnamon oil

2 tablespoons Epsom salt

2 tablespoons mango butter (cut into cubes and melt on its own before combining with the rest of the soap)

Directions:

Cut your base soap into smaller pieces, and melt with 1 teaspoon coconut oil in a pan on the stove. Stir often, until it is completely melted.

Add in the essential oils slowly, stirring the entire time. Remove from heat and set on a hot pad.

Keep an eye on the soap, and once it begins to harden, stir in any extra additive you wish to add. Let harden more, and once it is cool enough for you to handle it, form into the shape you desire.

Let sit for 24 hours, and your soap is done!

Perfect Moisture Body Soap

What you will need:

1 bar all natural base soap free of any additives

15 drops myrrh

10 drops lavender essential oil

Small handful dried lavender

1 tablespoon beeswax

1 teaspoon beet juice

Directions:

Cut your base soap into smaller pieces, and melt with 1 teaspoon coconut oil in a pan on the stove. Stir often, until it is completely melted.

Add in the essential oils slowly, stirring the entire time. Remove from heat and set on a hot pad.

Keep an eye on the soap, and once it begins to harden, stir in any extra additive you wish to add. Let harden more, and once it is cool enough for you to handle it, form into the shape you desire.

Let sit for 24 hours, and your soap is done!

Just Right Hand Soap

What you will need:

1 bottle clear hand soap (all natural variety)

15 drops myrrh

5 drops cinnamon

5 drops peppermint essential oil

5 drops vanilla essential oil

2 tablespoons water

Glass jar with pump for storage and use

Directions:

Pour your liquid soap into a glass bowl, and stir in the essential oils.

If you choose to add in any other extra, make sure they are very small... small enough to fit through the pump of the soap dispenser.

Stir these in, and add 1 to 2 teaspoons of water to achieve the desired consistency.

Pour into your soap dispenser, and you are set!

Behind Your Ears Body Wash

What you will need:

1 bottle liquid base soap, all natural and free of any kind of additives

1 teaspoon Epsom salt

1 teaspoon mango butter (completely melted before you add it to the soap)

1 teaspoon coconut oil

3 tablespoons water

20 drops spearmint essential oil

5 drops tea tree essential oil

Glass jar with pump for storage and use

Directions:

Pour the liquid base soap in a bowl.

Add in the essential oils, and the two tablespoons of water.

Break up the extra additions you are adding into your soap. You want body wash to be more a liquid than a solid, so the smaller the better with the extras.

Stir everything together, and pour into your dispenser.

That's it! Your new body wash is ready to spoil you whenever you are ready!

Conclusion

There you have it, everything you need to know to make your own soap, and to make it in the safest way you can imagine. I want everyone to be able to make soap, no matter how many small children they have at home, how little time they have to spend in the kitchen, or how much experience they have with crafts like this.

I know there are a lot of warnings and things you have to be aware of when you make soap in the traditional manner, and that you need to be especially careful of the lye. I know that this causes problems for the young and ambitious when they have little children at home that they need to take care of.

But, with this book, you can see that you can make your own soap in a single afternoon, and you can make it without using anything that is dangerous to yourself or anyone around you. The soaps that you find in this book are all entirely natural, but they are safe, and they get the job done.

Consider all of your gifting problems solved, and say goodbye to spending hours at the store trying to pick out that specific bar of soap you need for your particular needs. This book is going to take all of that away, and give you the freedom to make your own soap whenever you like, however you like.

So if you are ready to take the step into the all-natural realm, and get exactly what you want while you stay away from the things that you don't, you have come to the right place.

There's no better time than right now to start with this new hobby, and take your dream of making your own soap from an idea to a reality.

The entire world of soap making has been opened to you, all you have to do is jump on in and go for it.

Homemade Organic Sunscreen

Introduction

Summer is for lounging around by the pool, hitting the beach and going on holidays and let's be honest, for most of us the sun plays an important part in this. Everyone loves a sun tan which is a badge of pride that we have been somewhere warm and exotic and to many it is much more desirable. Women everywhere flock to the beach or even opt for synthetic spray tans or sun beds in the hopes of getting the illusive bronze look.

But what happens when you go too far? You get burnt. Many people don't realise that the sun can be just as damaging in the winter as it can in the summer and you need to protect your skin. Protecting your skin does not always mean you won't get a sun tan, but you must do it in the right way. Chapter 2 discussed what happens with regular unprotected exposure and the serious health implications.

Another common misconception is that you only need to apply sunscreen once and it will protect you. This is not true and is especially false for children who are generally in and out of the water or running around and rubbing off the protective layer. Kids are more susceptible to the negative impacts of the sun with as little as 2 hours unprotected midday sun can be life threatening if you do not properly protect them.

That being said, with the recipes in this eBook and the   knowledge that you gain, there is no reason why you and your family can't enjoy summer the right way while being completely and naturally protected as possible.

Chapter 1 – The Importance of Skin Care

The sun is a daily part of our lives, we go outside all the time and there is usually little need for applying sunscreen every day (unless you spend long hours in the sun specifically). Many people believe that because of the daily exposure to the sun, the body builds up a tolerance and therefore does not need special protection and this is partly true. While generally you acclimatize to the level of natural exposure in your country (for example, those in Australia have a higher tolerance to the sun and are less likely to get burned due to their constant exposure compared to elsewhere such as England) which means you are at a lower risk to get burned, that does not reduce the risk that sun damage can cause.

UV radiation is what causes most forms of skin cancer including melanoma which is the most serious and difficult to treat (see below). Those who are in sunny climates whether the climate is warm or not can put you at extra risk of skin damaged caused by the UV exposure. For example, many skiers have to apply vast amounts of sunscreen to avoid getting burnt even in the extremely cold temperatures because the UV is amplified and is incredibly direct in those areas (perfect for skiing, not for the skin.)

Sun and UV exposure affects everyone and that is why you should always apply sunscreen if you are going to be in the sun for a prolonged amount of time, regardless of the weather. Many people underestimate the effect that continuous and unrestricted UV radiation has on the body and can cause many health issues such as;

Premature Skin Aging – Repetitive exposure to UV radiation (including from sunbeds) causes the skin to lose its elasticity and therefore it starts to sag, specifically in the face. In addition to this, it can cause the skin to have a "leather" feel after hardening due to prolonged sun damage. Those who are frequently out in the sun may actually start to appear older because the collagen in the skin starts to break down and does not rejuvenate as easily causing more rapid aging. In addition, the sagging tends to lead to bags and wrinkles, specifically under the eyes and in the neck area which can give a more tired appearance.

Tumors – Although many tumors as a result of UV radiation are actually benign, this can still cause health implications and rapid growth of skin cells that are abnormal. While this can also lead to cancer, benign tumors that grow in the wrong areas can cause thyroid issues, affect body functions and even mood swings. Benign tumors are usually also removed to prevent further growth and this would require surgery that could otherwise have been avoided.

Longer healing time – Skin that has been exposed to vast amounts of UV radiation has a damaged immune function response which means that it struggles to repair itself quickly. This can cause higher risks for surgery patients or those with other medical conditions and it can create problems for something as simple as a cut that is unable to heal as quickly. In addition, the skin is the first line of defense for viruses and bacteria which is compromised with repeated, unprotected exposure and will leave you more open to colds and infections if not properly protected.

Pigment Discoloration – In some cases, UV radiation can cause what is called mottled pigmentation which results in the skin losing some of the melanin and not producing anymore which means that parts of the skin become a lot lighter than other areas which gives a "patchy" skin tone. While this is not threatening to your health, the areas with the lack of melanin that are lighter are more prone to burning in the sun and can develop other skin issues such as dry flakey skin or eczema.

<u>Skin Cancer</u> – This is the big one that many know about and due to the lowered immune system and the promotion of abnormal cell growth, UV radiation is the leading cause of skin cancer. 2 out of 3 types of skin cancer are less serious and can be easily treated however melanoma is the most serious. It is responsible for over 70% of skin cancer related deaths because it is the type that is able to spread to other body organs quickly and is difficult to regulate. Children that are sun burned are at a higher risk of developing melanoma in their adult lives due to damaging the growing cells and immune system from a young age. Those with lighter skin or red or blonde hair are also at a higher risk due to less melanin pigment naturally occurring in their skin and those with darker skin and hair have less risk.

Direct sunlight without protection can also cause an array of other problems from sun stroke to dehydration which can all be severely taxing on the body and in some cases even fatal (especially in children). Sun burn is also a high risk, especially if you are changing climates and are not used to the level of sun exposure that you will be receiving. Getting sun burn can send your body into shock in the same way you would if you were exposed to a flame and can not only be incredibly painful but can cause a range of health implications as well. If you have experienced sun burn, chapters 17-31 should contain the recipes to soothe and rejuvenate the skin and chapters 2-16 should be able to prevent this from happening in the future.

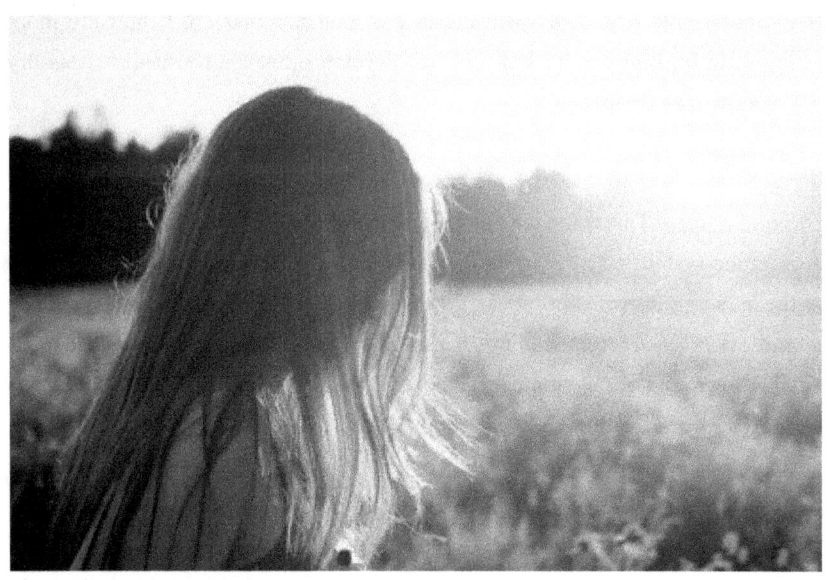

Chapter 2 – Jojoba Oil Sun cream

<u>You will need</u>

- 1 ounce of Coconut Oil

- Zinc Oxide Powder (follow instructions for quantities depending on brand)

- 0.1 Ounce of Jojoba Oil

- 1 Ounce of Shea Butter

- 1 ½ Tablespoons Eucalyptus Essential Oil

- 0.1 Ounce Vitamin E Oil

<u>Method</u>

1. Add the coconut oil, Shea butter and jojoba oil to a double boiler and melt gently together but do not allow to bubble.

2. Allow it to cool and add the vitamin E oil, essential oil and zinc powder to the mixture and stir together until all ingredients are combined.

3. Keep in the fridge in a darkened jar.

<u>Notes</u>:

Make sure to use a mask or protective equipment to avoid inhaling the zinc oxide powder.

<u>To Use</u>:

Apply to skin that is exposed to sunlight and make sure to use liberally and reapply frequently to maintain protection.

Chapter 3 - Almond Sunscreen

<u>You will need</u>

- 1 ounce of Coconut Oil

- Zinc Oxide Powder (follow instructions for quantities depending on brand)

- 0.1 Ounce of Sunflower Oil

- 0.8 Ounces of Almond Butter

- 0.1 Ounce Vitamin E Oil

<u>Method</u>

1. Add the coconut oil, almond butter and sunflower oil to a double boiler and melt gently together but do not allow to bubble.

2. Allow it to cool and add the vitamin E oil and zinc powder to the mixture and stir together until all ingredients are combined

3. Keep in the fridge in a darkened jar.

<u>Notes</u>:

- Make sure to use a mask or protective equipment to avoid inhaling the zinc oxide powder.

- Should Last approximately 6 months

<u>To Use</u>:

Apply to skin that is exposed to sunlight and make sure to use liberally and reapply frequently to maintain protection.

Chapter 4 – Lavender Sunscreen

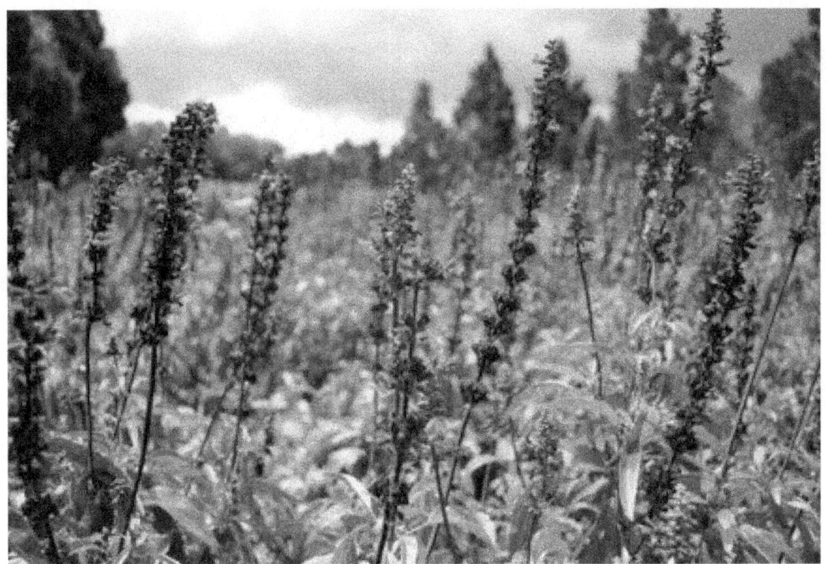

Photo Source: Free Stock Photo

<u>You will need</u>

½ Cup of Olive Oil

1/8 Cup Lavender Flower

¼ Cup of Beeswax

¼ Cup of Coconut Oil

2 Tablespoons Zinc Oxide Powder

1 Teaspoon Vitamin E Oil

1 ½ Tablespoons Lavender Essential Oil

<u>Method</u>

1. Infuse the olive oil and the lavender heads together and then strain when done to remove the excess plant material.

2. Add all of the ingredients (except the zinc oxide) into a double boiler and gently melt them together while stirring occasionally.

3. Remove from the heat and now add the zinc oxide powder

4. Stir and place in a jar or tin to store.

<u>Notes</u>:

- Use within 6 months

- Do not keep in direct sunlight

- Make sure to use a mask or protective equipment to avoid inhaling the zinc oxide powder.

Chapter 5 – Peppermint Oil Sun Cream

<u>You will need</u>

- ¼ Cup of Almond Oil

- ¼ Cup of Beeswax

- 2 Tbsp. Shea Butter

- 1 Tsp Peppermint Essential Oil

- 1 Tsp Carrot Seed Oil

- 2 Tablespoons Zinc Oxide Powder

- 1 Tsp Vitamin E Oil

- ¼ Cup of Coconut Oil

<u>Method</u>

1. Add the Shea butter, beeswax and almond oil to a double boiler and stir until completely melted.

2. Add the essential oil, carrot seed oil, vitamin E and coconut oil and stir further until completely mixed.

3. Remove from the heat and add the zinc oxide powder.

4. Transfer to darkened storage glass jars or tins

<u>Notes</u>:

- Use within 6 months

- Do not store in direct sunlight

- Refrigerate

- Make sure to use a mask or protective equipment to avoid inhaling the zinc oxide powder.

Chapter 6 – Soothing Eucalyptus Sunscreen

<u>You will need</u>

- 1 Teaspoon of Red Raspberry Seed Oil

- 2 Teaspoons Eucalyptus Oil

- ½ Cup Olive Oil

- ¼ Cup Shea Butter

- 2 Tablespoons Zinc Oxide Powder

- 1 Teaspoon Vitamin E Oil

- 1 Teaspoon Peppermint Essential Oil

- 2 Tablespoons Beeswax

<u>Method</u>

1. Add the Shea butter and beeswax to a double boiler and melt. (stir occasionally)

2. Add the oils and stir again until completely mixed

3. Remove from the heat and then add the zinc oxide powder. Stir until completely mixed.

4. Transfer to darkened storage containers.

<u>Notes</u>:

- Do not use in direct sunlight

- Make sure to use a mask or protective equipment to avoid inhaling the zinc oxide powder.

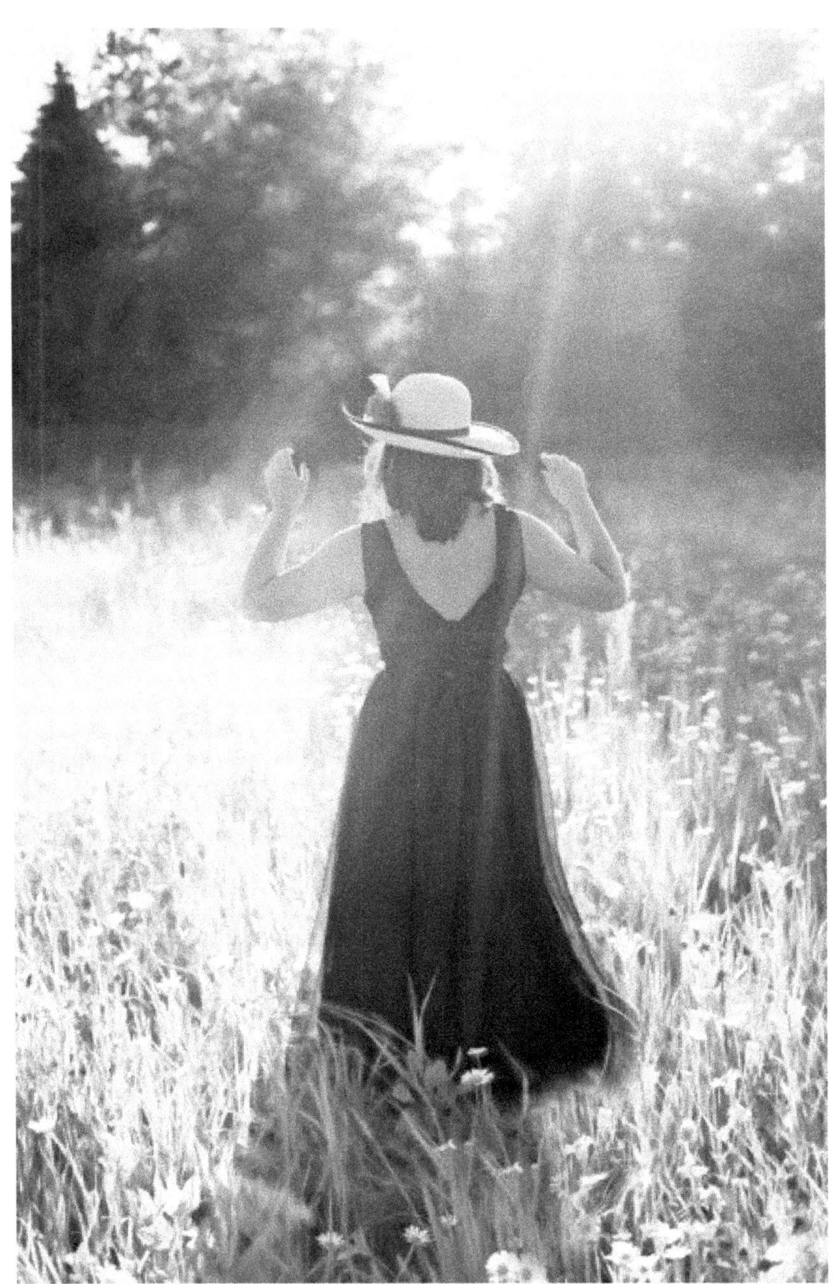

Photo Source: Free Stock Image

Chapter 7 – Pomegranate Shea Sun Cream

<u>You will need</u>

- 2 Tablespoons Shea Butter

- 1 Tablespoon Pomegranate Oil

- 2 Teaspoons Lavender Essential Oil

- 2 Tablespoons Zinc Oxide powder

- ¾ Cup Coconut Oil

<u>Method</u>

1. Using a double boiler, melt together the Shea butter and coconut oil and stir occasionally.

2. Stir in the pomegranate and lavender oil until completely mixed in.

3. Remove from the heat and add the zinc oxide powder making sure to carefully stir it in.

<u>Notes</u>:

- Store in a glass jar in the fridge

- Make sure to use a mask or protective equipment to avoid inhaling the zinc oxide powder.

Chapter 8– Natural Tinted Avocado Oil Sunscreen

<u>You will need</u>

- ¾ Cup Avocado Oil

- 3 Tbsp. Beeswax

- ¾ Cup Rose Water

- 2 Teaspoons Cocoa Powder (natural tinting agent)

- 3 Tablespoons Zinc Oxide Powder

- 1 Teaspoon Rose Essential Oil (optional)

<u>Method</u>

1. Add the avocado oil, beeswax and rose water to a double boiler and use a medium heat to mix all of the ingredients together, making sure to stir thoroughly.

2. Add the essential oil (if using) and mix together completely.

3. Remove from the heat and add the cocoa powder and zinc oxide powder to the mixture and stir until completely combined.

4. Allow to cool and store in the fridge.

<u>Notes</u>

Always use protective clothing or equipment when handling zinc oxide powder and do not inhale.

Chapter 9 – Coconut Grapeseed Oil Sunscreen

<u>You will need</u>

- 7 Ounces Grapeseed Oil

- 1 Ounce Coconut Oil

- 1.5 Ounces Beeswax

- 1 Teaspoon Coconut Essential Oil

- 2 Tablespoons Micronized Titanium Dioxide

<u>Method</u>

1. Using a double boiler, melt the beeswax, coconut oil and grapeseed oil together and mix until completely combined.

2. Add the essential oil and stir in thoroughly.

3. Remove the mixture from the heat and add the titanium dioxide, make sure to thoroughly stir in and mix all of the particles.

4. Allow to cool and store in a darkened glass jar.

<u>Notes</u>

- Make sure not to breathe in the titanium dioxide and wear protective clothing when handling as it can be an irritant.

Chapter 10– Beeswax Sunscreen with Vitamin E

<u>You will need</u>

- ½ Cup Coconut Oil

- 1/8 Cup Beeswax

- 1/8 Cup Shea Butter

- 1/3 Cup Jojoba Oil

- 3 Tablespoons Zinc Oxide Powder

- ½ Teaspoon Vitamin E Oil

<u>Method</u>

1, Using a double boiler, heat the coconut oil, beeswax and Shea butter together making sure that you mix occasionally.

2. Once combined, add the jojoba oil and vitamin E oil to the mixture and mix together completely.

3. Remove the mixture from the heat and stir in the zinc oxide powder thoroughly.

4. Allow to cool and store in a cool place.

<u>Notes</u>

- Make sure to use a mask or protective equipment to avoid inhaling the zinc oxide powder.

- Ensure to re-apply liberally to maintain protection

Chapter 11 – Coconut & Apricot Sunscreen

<u>You will need</u>

- ½ Cup Apricot Oil

- 1/8 Cup Beeswax

- 1/3 Cup Almond Oil

- 1/8 Cup Shea Butter

- 4 Tablespoons Zinc Oxide Powder

- 2 Teaspoons Coconut Oil

- ½ Teaspoon Coconut Essential Oil (optional)

<u>Method</u>

1. Place all of the ingredients (apart from the zinc oxide powder) into a bowl and heat using a double boiler.

2. Stir frequently until all of the ingredients are combined

3. Remove from the heat and carefully mix in the zinc oxide powder.

<u>Notes</u>

- Store in the refrigerator for no more than 6 months

- Make sure to use a mask or protective equipment to avoid inhaling the zinc oxide powder.

Photo Source: Free Stock Image

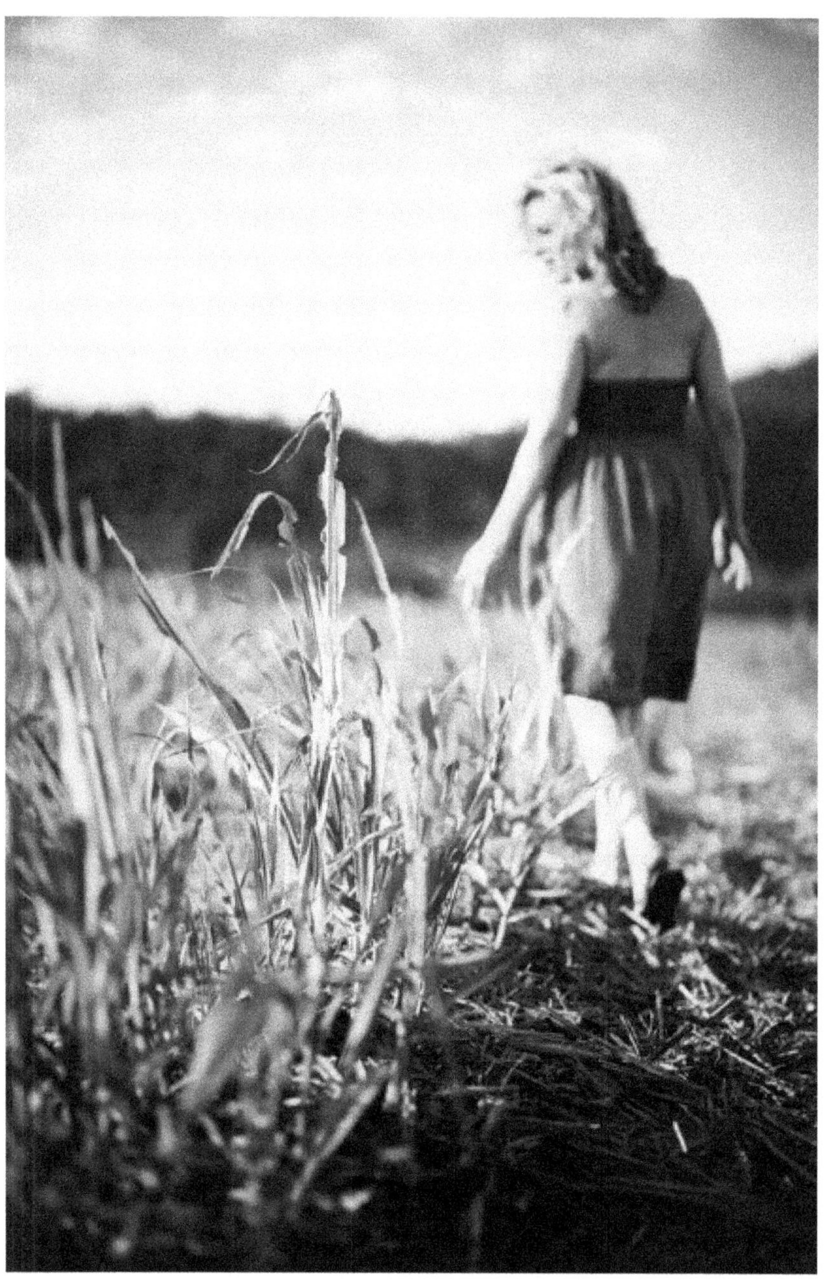

Chapter 12 – Mint and Shea Butter Sun Cream

<u>You will need</u>

- 1 Ounce Coconut Oil

- 1 Ounce of Olive Oil

- 1 Teaspoon Mint Leaves

- 1 Ounce Zinc Oxide Powder

- 2 Ounces Shea Butter

- ½ Teaspoon Peppermint Essential Oil

<u>Method</u>

1. Infuse the olive oil with the mint leaves by mixing them and leaving them overnight.

2. Strain the mixture and discard the plant material.

3. Add all of the ingredients to a double boiler (apart from the Zinc oxide) and mix together completely, making sure to stir frequently.

4. When completely combined, remove from the heat and gently stir in the zinc oxide powder.

5. Allow to cool and store in darkened jars.

<u>Notes</u>:

- Make sure to use a mask or protective equipment to avoid inhaling the zinc oxide powder.

Chapter 13 – Calendula Infused Sun Cream

<u>You will need</u>

- ½ Cup Olive Oil

- 4 Tablespoons Calendula

- ¼ Cup Coconut Oil

- 1/8 Cup Beeswax

- ½ Cup Shea Butter

- 1 Tsp Vitamin E Oil

- 2 Teaspoons Zinc Oxide Powder

<u>Method</u>

1. Infuse the calendula and olive oil by steeping the flowers overnight. In the morning remove the plant material.

2. Add the infused oil, beeswax, Shea butter and coconut oil to a double boiler and soften, mixing frequently.

3. Add the vitamin E oil and stir until mixed thoroughly.

4. Remove from the heat and carefully add the zinc oxide powder.

5. Transfer to storage jars and allow to completely cool before using.

<u>Notes:</u>

- Store for less than 6 months in the fridge

- Apply frequently and liberally

- Make sure to use a mask or protective equipment to avoid inhaling the zinc oxide powder.

Chapter 14– Sun Cream with Aloe Vera

You will need

- 1/8 Cup Avocado Oil

- 1/8 Cup Beeswax

- ¼ Cup Shea Butter

- ½ Cup Aloe Vera (the best format is gel)

- 2 Teaspoons Zinc Oxide Powder

- ½ Cup Coconut Oil

- 2 Teaspoons Lavender Essential Oil

Method

1. Add all of the ingredients to a double boiler except the zinc oxide powder and soften.

2. Stir frequently until all of the ingredients are completely mixed together.

3. Remove from the heat and stir in the zinc oxide powder until mixed in

4. Allow to cool and add to darkened glass jars

Notes:

- Store in the fridge

- Make sure to use a mask or protective equipment to avoid inhaling the zinc oxide powder.

Chapter 15 – Cocoa Butter Sunscreen

<u>You will need</u>

- ¼ Cup Cocoa Butter

- ¼ Cup Coconut Oil

- 1 ½ Teaspoons Red Raspberry Seed Oil

- 1/8 Cup Beeswax

- 1 Teaspoon Cocoa Powder (Optional for tint)

- 2 Teaspoons Zinc Oxide Powder

<u>Method</u>

1. Add the cocoa butter, beeswax and coconut oil to a double boiler and melt together thoroughly.

2. Stirring frequently add the raspberry seed oil and cocoa powder (if using) and stir until all the ingredients are thoroughly combined.

3. Take the mixture off of the heat and stir in the zinc oxide powder until thoroughly mixed and transfer to the storage tin or jar and allow to cool.

<u>Notes:</u>

- Store in a cool place

- Make sure to use a mask or protective equipment to avoid inhaling the zinc oxide powder.

Chapter 16 – Sesame and Coconut Sunscreen

<u>You will need</u>

- 1/8 Cup Olive Oil

- 1/8 Cup Neem Oil

- ¼ Cup Coconut Oil

- ¼ Cup Sesame Oil

- ¼ Cup Shea Butter

- 2 Teaspoons Zinc Oxide Powder

- 1 Teaspoon Vitamin E Oil

- 1 Teaspoon Eucalyptus Oil

- ¼ Cup Beeswax

<u>Method</u>

1. Add all of the ingredients to a double boiler except the zinc oxide powder and melt together making sure to stir frequently.

2. Once all of the ingredients are combined, remove the mixture from the heat and carefully add the zinc oxide power.

3. Stir it in completely and transfer to a darkened glass jar and store in the fridge.

<u>Notes</u>:

- Apply liberally and reapply every couple of hours

- Make sure to use a mask or protective equipment to avoid inhaling the zinc oxide powder.

After-Sun Recipes

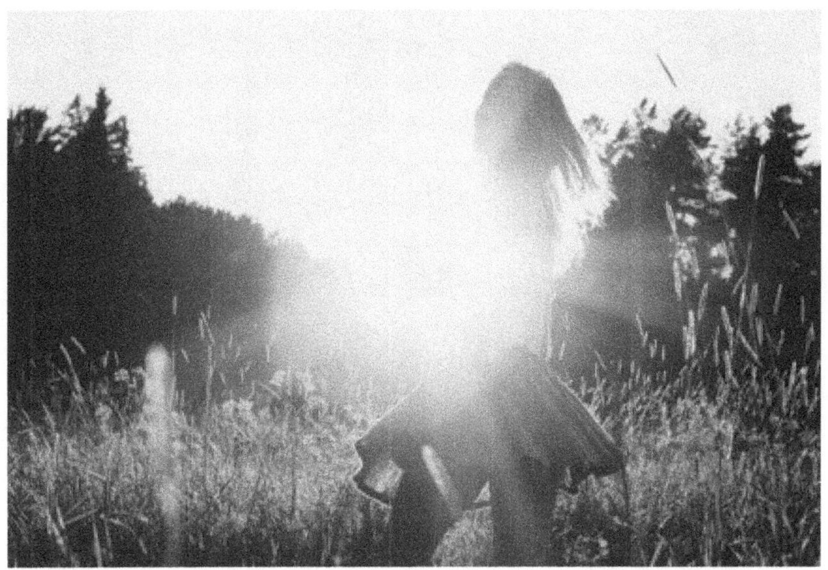

Photo Source: Free Stock Image

Chapter 17 – Aloe & Olive Oil After-Sun Lotion

<u>You will need</u>

- 1 Tbsp. Olive Oil

- 1 Tbsp. Shea butter

- 2 Tbsp. Coconut Oil

- 3 ½ Tbsp. Aloe Vera Gel

- 1 Teaspoon Eucalyptus Essential Oil

<u>Method</u>

1. Mix all of the ingredients in a bowl and stir until completely blended.

2. If the coconut oil or Shae butter is too hard you may need to warm it gently before mixing.

<u>Notes</u>

- Store in a darkened tin or glass jar

- Apply liberally

Chapter 18 – Cooling Peppermint After-sun Spray

<u>You will need</u>

- 4 Tablespoons Aloe Vera Gel

- Distilled Water

- 1 Tablespoon Apple Cider Vinegar (Raw)

- 6 Tablespoons Peppermint Hydrosol

- 2 Teaspoons Peppermint Essential Oil

- 8 Ounce Spray Bottle

- Optional: ½ Tablespoon Colloidal Silver (for extreme sunburn this helps to reduce infection)

<u>Method</u>

1. Mix all of the ingredients together and pour in the spray bottle.

2. Fill it up the rest of the way with the distilled water

3. Shake well and place in the fridge

<u>Notes</u>:

- Keep refrigerated

- Spray regularly to the affected area

- Avoid the eyes

- Do not use on children under 6

Chapter 19– Lavender Mist After-Sun Spray

<u>You will need</u>

- Distilled or purified water

- 1 Tablespoon Apple Cider Vinegar (Raw)

- 2 Teaspoons Lavender Oil

- 4 Tablespoons Aloe Vera Gel

- ½ Tablespoon Colloidal Silver

- ½ Tablespoon Vegetable Glycerin

- 8 Ounce Spray Bottle

<u>Method</u>

1. Add all of the ingredients to a bowl and mix thoroughly.

2. Pour into the spray bottle and top up with distilled or purified water.

3. Shake the bottle and refrigerate before using.

<u>Notes</u>:

- Do not spray in the eyes

- Keep refrigerated between uses

Chapter 20– Shea After-Sun Body Lotion

<u>You will need</u>

- 5 Tablespoons Shea Butter

- 1 Tablespoon Almond butter

- 3 Tablespoons Olive Oil

- 2 Tablespoons Aloe Vera Gel

- 1 Tablespoons Coconut Oil

<u>Method</u>

1. Add all of the ingredients into a bowl and stir until completely mixed.

2. Add to a storage container and leave in the fridge to allow it to gain some solidity

<u>Notes</u>

- You can use this recipe by itself or you can add it to your own organic body lotion and give it an extra boost.

- Use within 3-6 months

Chapter 21– Lavender & Aloe After-sun Oil

You will need

*   1 Teaspoon Lavender Blossom

*   2 Tablespoons Aloe Vera Gel

*   1 Teaspoon Lavender Essential Oil

*   3 Tablespoons Olive Oil

*   1 Tsp Cocoa Butter

*   1 Tsp Shea Butter

*   2 Tablespoons Beeswax

*   1 Teaspoon Coconut Oil

Method

1. Infuse the lavender blossom into the olive oil by steeping the flower overnight.

2. Drain and discard the leftover flowers.

3. Add the ingredients (including the infused olive oil) to a double boiler (except the Aloe Vera gel) and melt together until mixed.

4. Stir frequently and remove from the heat

5. Add the Aloe Vera gel and stir together thoroughly

6. Transfer to a container and store in the fridge

Notes:

Apply liberally and as regularly as needed

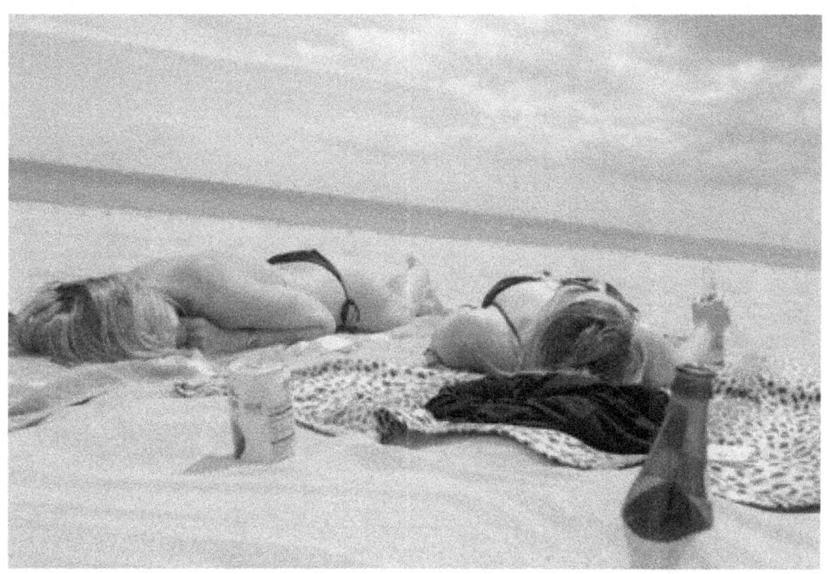

Photo Source: Free Stock Image

Chapter 22 – Calendula Butter After-Sun Oil

<u>You will need</u>

- 3 Tablespoons Olive Oil

- 1 Tablespoons Calendula Flowers

- 2 Tablespoons Cocoa Butter

- 2 Tablespoons Beeswax

- 2 Tablespoons Aloe Vera Gel

- 2 Teaspoons Eucalyptus Essential Oil

<u>Method</u>

1. Add the calendula flowers to the olive oil and vigorously stir for a few minutes.

2. Leave for an hour and then strain to remove the extra flowers

3. Add the butter and beeswax to a double boiler and heat until melted and mixed

4. Add the infused olive oil and essential oil to the mixture and stir completely

5. Remove from the heat and stir in the Aloe Vera gel

<u>Notes:</u>

- Store in the fridge in between uses

- Apply liberally to the affected area

Chapter 23 – Coconut & Eucalyptus After-Sun Lotion

<u>You will need</u>

- 4 Teaspoons Aloe Vera

- 4 Teaspoons Coconut Oil

- 1 Teaspoon Olive Oil

- 2 Teaspoons Shea Butter

- ½ Teaspoon Eucalyptus Essential Oil

<u>Method</u>

1. Add all of the ingredients into a bowl and beat together as you would with butter.

2. Combine all of the ingredients stir vigorously.

3. Place in a container and allow to set in the fridge overnight

<u>Notes</u>:

- Store in a cool, dry place

- Apply liberally

Chapter 24 – Olive Oil & Peppermint After-Sun Lotion

<u>You will need</u>

- 2 ½ Tablespoons Aloe Vera Gel

- 1 Tablespoon Almond Butter

- 1 Tablespoon Shea Butter

- 3 Tablespoons Olive Oil

- 1 Tablespoon Coconut Oil

- ½ Teaspoon Peppermint Essential Oil

<u>Method</u>

1. In a bowl, place all of the ingredients and beat together until smooth and creamy.

2. Transfer to a storage container and leave in a cool place. If you have a runnier texture then allow to set in the fridge overnight.

<u>Notes:</u>

- Apply topically whenever needed

Chapter 25 – Shea and Coconut After-sun Lotion

You will need

- 2 Tablespoons Shea Butter

- 3 Tablespoons Coconut Oil

- 2 ½ Tablespoons Aloe Vera

- 1 Teaspoon Lavender Essential Oil

- ½ Teaspoon Vitamin E Oil

- 1 Teaspoon Olive Oil

Method

1. Beat all of the ingredients together in a bowl and stir thoroughly until completely mixed.

2. Transfer to a storage container and leave in the fridge overnight to set

Notes

- Apply liberally every few hours on the affected area

Chapter 26 – Aloe & Witch Hazel After-Sun Spray

You will need

- 8 Tablespoons Fresh Aloe Pulp (from the plant)

- 5 Tablespoons Distilled Water

- 5 Tablespoons Witch Hazel

- ½ Teaspoon Eucalyptus Essential Oil

- 2 Tablespoons Vitamin E Oil

- 4 Ounce Spray bottle

Method

1. Combine the pulp, vitamin E and eucalyptus oil in a bowl and mix together thoroughly. Break apart any large clumps.

2. Pour the water and witch hazel into the mixture making sure to stir in completely.

3. Pour into the spray bottle and shake vigorously

Notes:

- Keep out of eyes

- Store in the fridge for extra cooling effect

- Will last 1-2 months

Photo Source: Free Stock Image

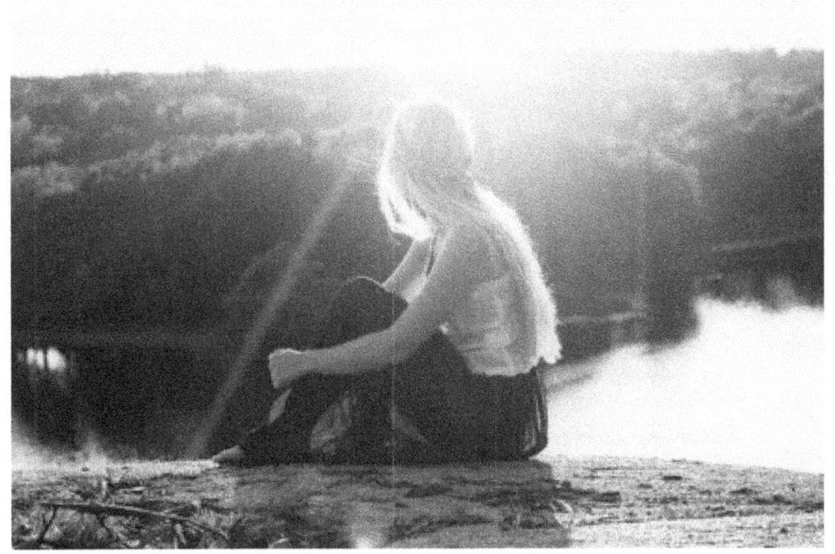

Chapter 27 – Chamomile After-Sun Lotion

<u>You will need</u>

- 2 Tablespoons St. John's Wort Oil

- 3 Tablespoons Olive Oil

- 2 Teaspoons Calendula Flowers

- 2 Tablespoons Chamomile Oil

- 1 Tablespoons Cocoa Butter

- 2 Tablespoons Beeswax

<u>Method</u>

1. Infuse the olive oil with the calendula flowers by stirring the two together and leaving them overnight.

2. Remove and discard the leftover plant material.

3. In a double boiler, melt together the cocoa butter, infused olive oil and beeswax, making sure to stir regularly until mixed together.

4. Add the St. John's Wort and chamomile oil and stir completely.

5. Allow to cool and transfer to a container and leave in the fridge

<u>Notes</u>:

- Apply liberally to affected area

- Store in the fridge and use within 2 months

Chapter 28 – Cocoa Butter & Rose After-Sun Lotion

<u>You will need</u>

- 2 Tablespoons Cocoa Butter

- 1 Tablespoon Beeswax

- 2 Tablespoons Aloe Vera Gel

- 2 Tablespoons Rose Water

- 1 Tablespoon Chamomile Oil

<u>Method</u>

1. Add all of the ingredients to a double boiler and gently heat until mixed together

2. Pour the mixture into a storage container and place in the fridge overnight to set before using.

<u>Notes</u>:

- Keep refrigerated

- Use within 1-2 months

Chapter 29 – Lavender & Witch Hazel After-Sun Spray

<u>You will need</u>

- 8 Tablespoons Aloe Vera Gel

- 1 ½ Teaspoons Lavender Essential Oil

- 2 Tablespoons Vitamin E Oil

- 4 Tablespoons Witch Hazel

- 6 Tablespoons Distilled or Purified Water

- 4 Ounce Spray Bottle

<u>Method</u>

1. Add the aloe gel, lavender and vitamin E oils to a bowl and stir together

2. Combine the witch hazel and stir into the mixture

3. Pour into the spray bottle and top up the rest with the distilled water

4. Shake vigorously and store in the fridge overnight before use.

<u>Notes</u>:

- Keep in the fridge for a cooling effect

- Keep out of eyes

- Use to soothe sunburnt skin

Chapter 30 – Simple 3 Ingredient After-sun Oil

<u>You will need</u>

- 2 Tablespoons Almond Oil

- ½ Teaspoon Eucalyptus Essential Oil

- 2 Tablespoons Almond Oil

- Spray Bottle

<u>Method</u>

1. Add all of the ingredients into the spray bottle and vigorously shake.

2. Keep in the fridge for an extra cooling effect

<u>Notes</u>

- Keep out of the eyes

- There is no need to wash this spray off, just allow it to soak into the skin naturally

Chapter 31 – Regeneration After-sun Butter

<u>You will need</u>

- 1 Tablespoon Shea Butter

- 1 Tablespoon Avocado Butter

- 2 Tablespoons Aloe Vera Pulp

- 1 Tablespoon Evening Primrose Oil

- 2 Teaspoons Eucalyptus Oil

- 1 Teaspoon Vitamin E Oil

<u>Method</u>

1. Add all of the ingredients into a bowl and beat together thoroughly. You may find you need to gently heat them to mix properly.

2. Once stirred and completely combined, transfer to a storage container and leave in the fridge overnight before the first use.

<u>Notes:</u>

- Store in the fridge

- Apply liberally and frequently to the affected area

Photo Source: Free Stock Image

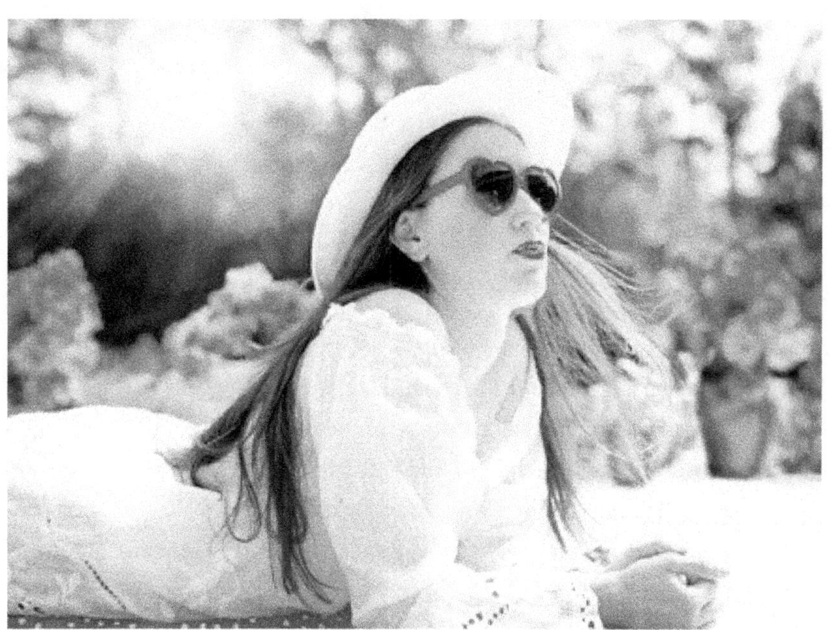

Conclusion

Hopefully this eBook has given you all the insight you need into the best ways to naturally protect yourself and your family from the sun. Using these recipes you can be safe in the knowledge that you can enjoy the sunshine and summer without any of the detrimental health risks. In addition to this you no longer have to be concerned about the chemicals that you exposing to yourself and family due to the commercial products on the market. You can also enjoy experimenting with these recipes to find the right texture, fragrance and protection that is right for you and you can easily adapt them for larger or smaller families. Finally, don't fall prey to the sun and enjoy it while being thoroughly protected.

Thanks for reading.

20 Herbs to use for Herbal Remedies to Maximize Your Health and Healing

Introduction

If you let yourself get caught up in the modern day world, you are going to find that you get pills and prescriptions shoved in your face for every single thing you feel. Whether you have a bad day, a bad cough, or a bad case of the sneezes, you are going to get someone shoving their bottle of pills toward you, expecting you to take it and use it to cure yourself.

The only issue is that you may not want to take these pills for a number of reasons. So many times synthetic pills bring on their own sets of problems. So many times you have to be careful of the pills you are taking or you could get worse, so many times you don't have the money to go spend on a prescription drug that is full of side effects.

If you care about doing things the natural way, odds are you will want to try to heal yourself with herbs. Sure, you may not be able to make anything go away completely, but then again, neither can the synthetic medications we see on the shelves today.

A lot of the time, you can heal or alleviate your symptoms by knowing where the solutions are in nature, and going with that. For thousands of years, mankind has been treating illness and symptoms with plants and herbs. No matter what kind of illness you had, you were able to find something for it in the herbal world.

Today, I am all about the herbal. The more natural you can live your life, the better. It is better for the environment, it is better for your wallet, and it is better for you not to put into your body all of those nasty chemicals they create in the lab.

When you use this book, you are going to find the simple and easy solution to your health needs, and you will be surprised to find that they are all around you. Grow some in your garden, buy dried versions at your grocery store. Wherever you want, pick up some of these herbs and put them to use.

You can prevent, treat, and even cure some of the most common ailments that like to plague your world, giving you that leg up on your day that you are always looking for. So if you are ready to step out of the synthetic world and take hold of the natural remedies, look no further.

This book has just what you need.

Chapter 1 – Getting Started

I know if you have been studying or if you have had any interest in herbal medication you are likely eager to jump in and see what this is all about. I am going
to show you the first few herbs you should have on hand at all times in just a
moment, but first, there are a few things I wanted to point out.

First of all, herbs are plants, and while you can use the herbs themselves, there
are always cautions to keep in mind when you are using plants, especially if
you have small children. Make sure you keep your herbs out of reach of small
children, and that you use them cautiously.

Always apply to children yourself, and never let them use them unsupervised.

In addition to this, you do need to realize that while herbs used as medication
don't have the same kinds of side effects synthetic medications do, you still
need to be aware that there are side effects involved to an extent, and there are
things you will need to watch out for.

If you are using any prescription medications right now, discuss with your doctor what your options are before you start. This is going to drastically reduce
any chance of bad interactions or overdose.

Insider's tip:

Yes, it is possible to overdose on herbs, just as it is other medications, so you need to keep them out of reach of children at all times. Watch for adverse side effects, and stop using them if you see any take place.

I am going to list the side effects along with the herbs that I list, so you know exactly what to watch out for.

So with those things in mind, we are ready to get started! Here are the first five herbs on the list. In the chapters to come we are going to add on more herbs.

Calendula

Use: Usually used topically, this is a great herb to use for sores in the mouth, throat, or stomach. It has been used for centuries with excellent results.

Preparation: wrap 2 teaspoons of leaves in a tea steeper and pour boiling water over the top. Let steep for 15 minutes, then remove the steeper. Gargle for 60 seconds. Repeat twice daily.

Things to watch for: There are no bad side effects from this herb

Catnip

Use: Not just for our feline friends, catnip has long been used to treat tension, anxiety, and as a calming agent for those that are high strung or just want to relax a bit at the end of the day.

Preparation: wrap 2 teaspoons of leaves in a tea steeper and pour boiling water over the top. Let steep for 15 minutes, then remove the steeper. Enjoy as tea twice daily.

Things to watch for: There are no bad side effects from this herb

Hibiscus

Use: this is a highly effective herb when it comes to lowering blood pressure. Other uses include soothing anxiety and promoting relaxation

Preparation: wrap 2 teaspoons of leaves in a tea steeper and pour boiling water over the top. Let steep for 15 minutes, then remove the steeper. Enjoy as tea twice daily.

Things to watch for: if you are taking this to help lower your high blood pressure, make sure you visit with your doctor and monitor where your blood pressure is at. Always keep an eye on it to ensure things are going as they should.

Garlic

Use: very powerful antimicrobial. It can also be used to lower blood pressure, and to treat colds and the flu.

Preparation: wrap 2 teaspoons of leaves in a tea steeper and pour boiling water over the top. Let steep for 15 minutes, then remove the steeper. Enjoy as tea twice daily.

Use in foods you prepare.

Apply topically to the infected area.

Things to watch for: May interact with certain medications such as warfarin

Elderberry

Use: Let this be your go to herb if you are dealing with a cold, fever, or the flu. Any and all of those symptoms will be taken care of with this charming herb.

Preparation: wrap 2 teaspoons of leaves in a tea steeper and pour boiling water over the top. Let steep for 15 minutes, then remove the steeper. Enjoy as tea twice daily.

Things to watch for: Using too much may result in an upset stomach, but there is nothing severe. Simply cut back on the amount you are using

Chapter 2 – Easy Elegant Herbs

Some of these herbs may surprise you, as they sound more like spices and treats than they do herbs, but you are going to find that these things we already use and love are actually powerful herbs that have incredible healing powers.

At the same time, you still need to be aware of the amount you are eating, and how often you are taking it. Make sure you read the entire description for any herb you decide to take, use it properly, and follow the directions.

This way, you are going to get the incredible benefits, but none of the adverse side effects I am helping you avoid.

Cranberries

Use: Use primarily for the urinary tract, this is the herb to turn to if you are feeling uncomfortable with infections or inflammations alike.

Preparation: wrap 2 teaspoons of leaves in a tea steeper and pour boiling water over the top. Let steep for 15 minutes, then remove the steeper. Enjoy as tea twice daily.

Things to watch for: There are no bad side effects from this herb

Ginger

Use: Ginger has often been sought out for its ability to cure an upset stomach, to rid the body of nausea, and to soothe aches and pains in the stomach.

Preparation: wrap 2 teaspoons of leaves in a tea steeper and pour boiling water over the top. Let steep for 15 minutes, then remove the steeper. Enjoy as tea twice daily.

Can be used to season foods as well.

Things to watch for: safe in small amounts. Too much can cause heartburn and upset stomach. Use carefully if you are pregnant.

Lavender

Use: lavender is the herb to have on hand if you deal with anxiety, insomnia, sleeplessness, or tension. This herb is one of the most powerful you can use to calm down and promote healthy sleep.

Preparation: wrap 2 teaspoons of leaves in a tea steeper and pour boiling water over the top. Let steep for 15 minutes, then remove the steeper. Pour the contents into the bath water of a hot bath, sit back, and enjoy.

Things to watch for: There are not any health concerns associated with the use of lavender, but as always, use in moderation and make sure you supervise children as they use it.

Hops

Use: hops is largely used for its calming effect on the body. Use this when you are feeling tight, anxious, or sleepless.

Preparation: wrap 2 teaspoons of leaves in a tea steeper and pour boiling water over the top. Let steep for 15 minutes, then remove the steeper. Enjoy as tea twice daily.

Can also be used in bath water

Things to watch for: Too much of this herb may cause sedation, and too much beyond that can prove to cause some real problems, make sure you use in moderation.

Peppermint

Use: This is truly a miracle herb, and as soon as you try it out for yourself, you are going to agree. There are few things you can't solve with a bit of peppermint, including stomach aches and pains, join pain, inflammation, headaches, heartburn, tension, and insomnia, just to name a few.

Preparation: wrap 2 teaspoons of leaves in a tea steeper and pour boiling water over the top. Let steep for 15 minutes, then remove the steeper. Enjoy as tea twice daily.

You can also soak a washcloth in the tea mixture and apply the washcloth to your forehead, your stomach, or anywhere you need pain relief.

Can also be poured into the bath for relaxation.

Things to watch for: too much peppermint can cause stomach pains. Use in moderation

Chapter 3 – Herbs for Most Anything

I greatly enjoy fresh herbs, and I highly condone growing them yourself, which is why I included a chapter at the end of the book on how to grow these herbs in your own home, but I also wanted you to be aware that you can find many of these herbs in capsule form in your local stores.

There are great benefits to this, as you can have the dosage you need, in a convenient little capsule that you can take at your leisure. Of course, you don't get quite the same benefits that you would get if you were using fresh herbs in your tea, but you are going to get the benefits to an extent.

If your option is capsule form, then I highly suggest you go that route rather than taking the other synthetic medication they try to offer you on the shelves.

Horse chestnuts

Use: a cosmetic herb, this is the herb you want to go to for varicose veins or anything along those lines. Watch your skin reclaim its youthful glow for good!

Preparation: wrap 2 teaspoons of leaves in a tea steeper and pour boiling water over the top. Let steep for 15 minutes, then remove the steeper. Enjoy as tea twice daily.

Can also mix the herb in with your lotion and apply to your arms and legs. You will need to rinse to get the solids off of you.

Things to watch for: too much of this herb, especially in its unprocessed form can prove to be toxic. Always use in extreme moderation, and use the best quality that you can get.

Ginseng

Use: this is the energizing herb, and you can find it when you need that bit of a boost in the afternoon. It is also known to help with the symptoms associated with the cold and flu, or even allergies.

Preparation: wrap 2 teaspoons of leaves in a tea steeper and pour boiling water over the top. Let steep for 15 minutes, then remove the steeper. Enjoy as tea twice daily.

Things to watch for: Ginseng is fine in moderation, if you are using a pure form of the herb. To ensure you get unadulterated herb, only purchase from a reputable supplier.

Kava

Use: This herb is terrific for anxiety, and has been known to help ward off even the worst of panic attacks. Keep some on hand, especially if you have to deal with panic attacks or stress often.

Preparation: wrap 2 teaspoons of leaves in a tea steeper and pour boiling water over the top. Let steep for 15 minutes, then remove the steeper. Enjoy as tea twice daily.

Things to watch for: too much of this herb has been known to cause toxicity in the liver. Use carefully, especially if you drink alcohol or take medications that can be hard on your liver.

Licorice

Use: this is one of the best anti-inflammatories you will ever set eyes on. Perfect for the mucous membranes, especially during illness. Use in moderation.

Preparation: wrap 2 teaspoons of leaves in a tea steeper and pour boiling water over the top. Let steep for 15 minutes, then remove the steeper. Enjoy as tea twice daily.

Take note, this is an herb that will build up in your system over time, so only use for a week at a time, then take a break for a few weeks. This isn't the same as the candy, and you can end up with new health problems if you aren't careful with your dosages.

Things to watch for: this herb builds up in your system through prolonged use, and you can take too much at a time. It causes high blood pressure, which you know can lead to dozens of other health problems or even death. Use cautiously.

Lemon Balm

Use: soothing, this is the herb to go to if you or your child is suffering from colic, upset stomach, fever, or tension

Preparation: wrap 2 teaspoons of leaves in a tea steeper and pour boiling water over the top. Let steep for 15 minutes, then remove the steeper. Enjoy as tea twice daily.

Can mix powdered form in lotion and massage into your skin as well.

Try using it in creams to soothe blisters and scrapes.

Things to watch for: there is nothing in this herb that will cause any problems for anyone, you can keep this on hand for everyone of all ages, and in any stage of life.

Chapter 4 – The Best of the Rest

You are likely wondering if these herbs interact with medications, if they may interact with each other. While they may to an extent, you don't have to worry about crossing them the same way you do medications.

On the other hand, you can use this to your advantage, because you can blend several herbs in a single tea or in a bath to reap the most of the benefits. As I have said before, everything in moderation, so be careful as you use your herbs, but also enjoy them, and use them for the benefits they offer.

You are going to be so glad that you did.

Marshmallow

Use: this coats the lining of your mouth and throat, making it the perfect go to herb for colds, sore throats, and the flu. Any agitation in the throat, this is your cure right here!

Preparation: wrap 2 teaspoons of leaves in a tea steeper and pour boiling water over the top. Let steep for 15 minutes, then remove the steeper. Enjoy as tea twice daily.

You don't have to worry about long term effects with this one, enjoy as many days as you would like.

Things to watch for: while there is nothing in this herb that is going to cause any damage of itself, you do need to be aware that this herb will slow your body's ability to absorb other medications. Be aware of how you use it.

Slippery Elm

Use: not only does this herb have a charming name, but it also has what you need if you are dealing with coughs, aches or pains. In essence, if you are having any allergy symptoms, or if you are dealing with a cold, brew up a batch and enjoy not only the flavor, but the relief that it brings.

Preparation: wrap 2 teaspoons of leaves in a tea steeper and pour boiling water over the top. Let steep for 15 minutes, then remove the steeper. Enjoy as tea twice daily.

You can also use this in your bath water as a soak.

Things to watch for: while you don't need to worry too much about this one, this herb has been known to slow the absorption of oral medications taken within a couple of hours of using this herb. Make sure you know when you are going to take any medications, and plan accordingly.

Milk Thistle

Use: This herb is said to be an excellent herb for detox. Use it for regular cleanses, and make sure you don't drink as you use it, or you aren't going to get the benefits that you are after.

Preparation: wrap 2 teaspoons of leaves in a tea steeper and pour boiling water over the top. Let steep for 15 minutes, then remove the steeper. Enjoy as tea twice daily.

If you can only find the capsule form, take a single serving daily.

Things to watch for: there aren't any known adverse side effects with Milk Thistle, but as with anything, it is important that you watch how you feel as you take it. Make adjustments as necessary.

Sage

Use: not only this this herb good for sore throat, coughing, and aches and pains, it is great for menopausal symptoms as well as PMS symptoms. Keep some on hand for that time of the month, or anytime you need a bit of relief.

Preparation: wrap 2 teaspoons of leaves in a tea steeper and pour boiling water over the top. Let steep for 15 minutes, then remove the steeper. Enjoy as tea twice daily.

Can also be added to food for seasoning, or you can find it in capsule form.

If you are taking capsules, follow the recommended dosage on the bottle.

Things to watch for: the leaves are fine to turn into tea, but you don't want to ingest the essential oil from this herb to use it. Also avoid using it during pregnancy. Moderation in all things, including this herb.

Nettle

Use: Used to relieve itchy eyes, scratching throat, and runny nose, this is the perfect herb to turn to for allergy symptoms any time of the year.

Preparation: wrap 2 teaspoons of leaves in a tea steeper and pour boiling water over the top. Let steep for 15 minutes, then remove the steeper. Enjoy as tea twice daily.

The water can also be added to bath water for a soak.

Things to watch for: you can use this herb as often as you like, there aren't any worries there, but you do need to make sure you wear gloves as you handle the herb, or you may end up with thorns in your fingers.

Chapter 5 – How Does Your Garden Grow?

When it comes to the topic of herbal remedies, you are going to want to have the freshest and best available. Of course, as you saw, you can use dried, story purchased, or pretty much any form of the herb you would like, but I still recommend that you use fresh herbs as much as you can.

That is why I have chosen to include this chapter, where you will find how you can grow your own herbs and keep them year round, constantly providing yourself with a source of fresh herbs for anything that comes your way.

I know not everyone has a green thumb, and the concept of growing your own garden can be daunting, no matter what kind of garden it is. Trust me, I know what it is like to watch your plants shrivel up and die in spite of your best efforts, which is why I have put together the method for any planter.

This is all you need to grow your own plants year round, no matter what kind of climate you live in, or how good you are at growing a garden.

For this garden you will need:

Large herbal pot (you can get this in stores usually in the spring or summer, but if you can't find one Amazon has them available)

Potting soil

Watering can

Paper markers

Pen

Herbs

Large plate (and a room that gets direct sunlight)

To assemble your garden you need to:

Fill your pot with the potting soil. You can see by the directions how to fill each of the individual pockets in the pot, or you can use a single spaced pot and fill this to the top with the soil, too.

Whichever you prefer.

If you live in a warmer climate, you can keep your herbs outdoors year round, but if you are in cooler climates, you will need to bring them in several months of the year. Even if you do live where it is warm, there are benefits to keeping your pot indoors as this is going to minimize the bugs and other nuisances that hinder the plant growth.

Once you have the spot picked out, place your pot on your plate, to catch any of the water that drains out of the pot.

Set markers in the pot, with the name of the herbs written on the marker. This way you are going to know which herbs are which in your pot, or you will be able to find the row you want if you are looking for something specific.

Plant the seeds, and water them daily.

Herbs are easy to grow, but they do require diligence. You are going to need to make sure the water stays moist, that your plants get exposure to sunlight daily, but that they don't scorch. One of the problems and common mistakes first time growers make is that they give their plants too much sunlight.

This ends up working against them as the plants get too hot and burn, ruining the herbs. Make sure your plants get the morning sun, but that they are also out of the direct sunlight by noon. If you need, and if you are able, you can always move the pot into the shade as the day wears on, just make sure you are consistent with this.

That's really all you need to do, the rest of the time you are going to spend watching and weeding. Even the most well kept garden (including the ones indoors) can get weeds in them from time to time. This happens because the seeds can get stuck in clothing, fur, or blow in through an open door or window.

Simply keep an eye on the plants, take out the plants that shouldn't be there, and thin them out as you need to.

If you are consistent with this, you are going to see your herbs mature into grown plants.

Once your herbs are grown, you can harvest them and use them time and time again.

In other words, don't get overly excited when you harvest your herbs. Pull some of the leaves off, next to the stem.

Use these in whatever way you need, and keep caring for the rest of the plant as you would if you hadn't taken any of the leaves. In as little as a few days, you are going to notice new growth coming in, and in no time at all the leaves are going to replace themselves.

Space out your usage and care for the plant, letting the new leaves mature before you use them, and you are going to keep your system going for as long as you need.

Have fun with it, and don't stress that you can't get them to grow at first. The more consistent you are with your plants, and the more you pay attention to them, the better you are going to be able to give them what they need.

Practice makes perfect, and in no time at all you are going to have everything you need to sustain your herbal healing.

Conclusion

There you have it, everything you need to know about the herbs you need to treat and cure any of the illnesses that plague you. You will find that it doesn't matter what happens, you are going to have what you need on hand at all times, and never have to worry about that annoying headache or painful stomach ache again.

This book is exactly what you need to make your home remedies complete, and take away all of the guesswork that comes with herbal remedies. I know when you are first starting, you wonder just what you can and can't have, or what you should and shouldn't use for the symptoms you are feeling, but this book is going to take away all of that, and get you on the right track where you should be.

I hope you are now able to see what you need to cure and treat all of the symptoms you feel, and that you are able to see how easy it is to get these things, or even grow them in your home.

All you need is a few seeds, a place to set them up, and some time on your hands, and with minimal care, you are going to be able to grow your own garden of health. You will find that everything you need is so easy to grow and inexpensive to purchase, you will wonder why you have never done this before.

This book holds the secret you need to having complete success with at home remedies. You are going to find everything from what kinds of plants you need to how to use the herbs to alternate ways of using them. You will see just how easy it is to grow them yourself, and get your own herbal garden going.

In no time at all, you are going to have everything right at your fingertips, making any ailment or any symptom a thing of the past. No more worry about what prescriptions you may need, no more wondering how you are going to pay for them, and no more stressing that they are going to interact with the medication you are already taking.

When you use plants to heal yourself, you are going to the source. The completely natural remedy that has been around for thousands of years, and that has stood the test of time. No stress that it isn't going to work, no wondering if you are going to need to refill the prescription, and no more stressing that you don't have enough or that you took too much.

This book is your key to success, and in it you are going to get just what you need to treat anything that comes your way. Use this book with confidence, knowing that you are getting just what you need to treat anything you want to treat. It is going to be fast, easy, and inexpensive. The best of both worlds.

FREE Bonus Reminder

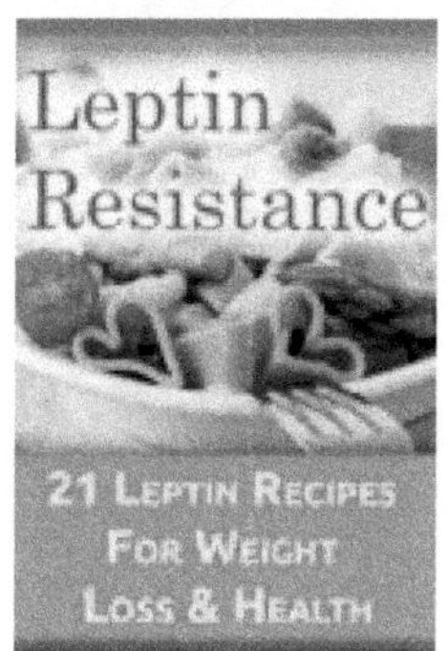

If you have not grabbed it yet, please go ahead and download your special bonus report *"Leptin Resistance. 21 Leptin Recipes For Weight Loss & Healthy Living"*.

Simply Click the Button Below

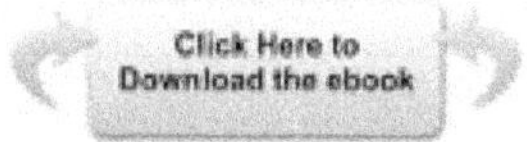

OR **Go to This Page**

http://easyweightlossway.com/free/

BONUS #2: More Free & Discounted Books

Do you want to receive more Free & Discounted Books?

We have a mailing list where we send out our new Books when they go free or with a discount on Kindle. Click on the link below to sign up for Free & Discount Book Promotions.

=> Sign Up for Free & Discount Book Promotions <=

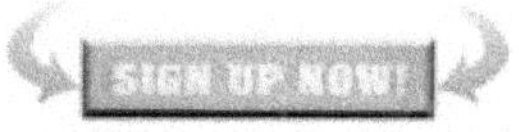

OR Go to this URL

http://zbit.ly/1WBb1Ek